APPLIED THIRD EDITION
KNOWLEDGE
TEST FOR THE MRCGP

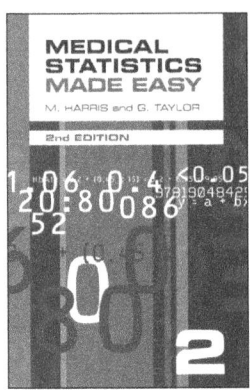
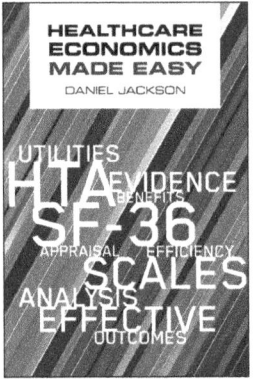
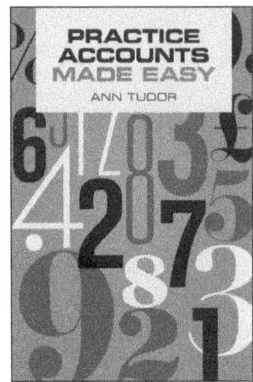
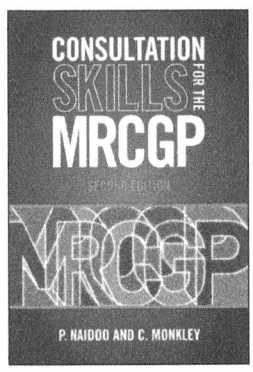
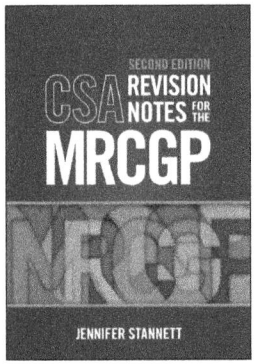
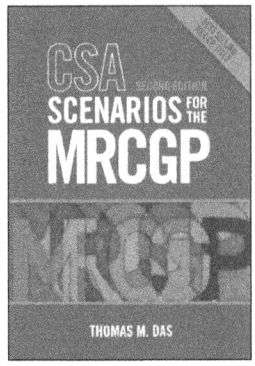
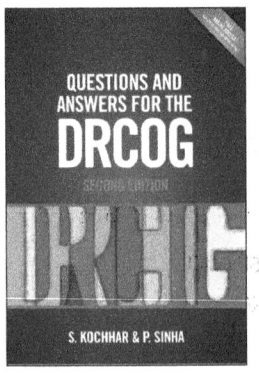
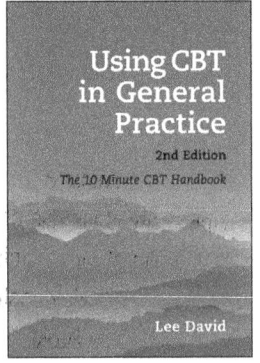
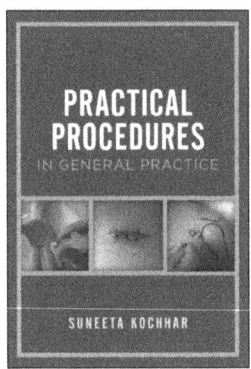
For more details see www.scionpublishing.com

APPLIED THIRD EDITION
KNOWLEDGE
TEST FOR THE MRCGP

QUESTIONS AND ANSWERS FOR THE AKT

NUZHET A-ALI
MBBS, MRCGP, DRCOG, DFFP, DCH
GP Trainer in Berkshire

Scion

© **Scion Publishing Limited, 2014**

ISBN 978 1 907904 18 9

Third edition first published 2014

Second edition published 2010, reprinted 2013

A CIP catalogue record for this book is available from the British Library.

Scion Publishing Limited

The Old Hayloft, Vantage Business Park, Bloxham Road, Banbury OX16 9UX, UK

www.scionpublishing.com

Important Note from the Publisher

The information contained within this book was obtained by Scion Publishing Ltd from sources believed by us to be reliable. However, while every effort has been made to ensure its accuracy, no responsibility for loss or injury whatsoever occasioned to any person acting or refraining from action as a result of information contained herein can be accepted by the authors or publishers.

Readers are reminded that medicine is a constantly evolving science and while the authors and publishers have ensured that all dosages, applications and practices are based on current indications, there may be specific practices which differ between communities. You should always follow the guidelines laid down by the manufacturers of specific products and the relevant authorities in the country in which you are practising.

Although every effort has been made to ensure that all owners of copyright material have been acknowledged in this publication, we would be pleased to acknowledge in subsequent reprints or editions any omissions brought to our attention.

Registered names, trademarks, etc. used in this book, even when not marked as such, are not to be considered unprotected by law.

Typeset by Phoenix Photosetting, Chatham, Kent, UK

Printed in the UK

Contents

Preface

Since the second edition of this book in 2010, the Applied Knowledge Test continues to be an integral part of the MRCGP licensing exam.

This new edition has been produced to help candidates prepare for this exam and contains over 450 questions. These aim to cover the exam curriculum and reflect the format of the actual exam using single best answer, extended matching questions, rank ordering, picture format and algorithm completion question types.

It has been favourably reviewed by trainees, trainers and programme directors alike and is on the recommended reading lists of a number of VTS schemes, making it essential not only for candidates sitting the AKT but also for training practices and libraries. It has been used by trainers to plan teaching sessions and tutorials and by established GPs to help them with appraisal and revalidation.

As a trainer I can appreciate there are a huge number of websites dedicated to the AKT and I would advise candidates to practise as many questions as they can; however, with its portability and convenient sections of fifty questions at a time, the 'Applied Knowledge Test for the MRCGP' means learning can easily be slotted into a busy working day and be used to supplement online revision.

The questions continue to be grounded in everyday practice and are based on feedback from the Royal College on the performance of candidate in recent sittings of the exam. Areas most recently identified as causing difficulty for candidates include:

- skin lesions
- dermatology – safe prescribing
- contraception including LARC
- screening programmes – antenatal and general
- management of childhood asthma
- child health – normal range of developmental milestones and immunisations
- drug doses and calculations
- side-effects of commonly used drugs
- controlled drug regulations
- osteoporosis
- diabetes – interpreting diagnostic test results

The new questions have therefore been written with these comments in mind.

Questions have also been added or revised to reflect changes since the last edition in management of clinical areas such as generalised anxiety disorder, hypertension, fertility, ectopic pregnancy, atrial fibrillation and the early management of ovarian cancer and Alzheimer's disease as well as in administrative areas such as the new fit notes with references updated throughout.

I do hope this revision aid helps you in your journey to becoming independent practitioners. This book is dedicated to my trainees, who continue to make training such a pleasure and a privilege.

Dr Nuzhet A-Ali
August 2013

Acknowledgements

I would like to thank the reviewers of early drafts of this book: Dr Julia Fisher, Dr Penny Halls, Dr Craig Mason, Dr Kate Roberts-Lewis, and Dr Lisa Burton for their helpful comments and critiques.

Introduction

Since August 2007 there has been a single training and assessment system for UK-trained doctors wishing to obtain a Certificate of Completion of Training (CCT) in General Practice. Satisfactory completion of the scheme is an essential requirement for entry to the General Medical Council's GP Register and for membership of the Royal College of General Practitioners. The MRCGP is an integrated assessment programme that includes three components:

- Applied Knowledge Test (AKT)
- Clinical Skills Assessment (CSA)
- Workplace-Based Assessment (WPBA)

Each of these is independent and tests different skills, but together they cover the curriculum for specialty training for general practice. Evidence for the workplace-based assessment is collected in the e-portfolio of each GP trainee.

This book is intended to help candidates identify learning needs, prioritise learning and target revision by practising questions with a view to passing the AKT component of the MRCGP.

The AKT

The AKT is a summative assessment of the knowledge base that underpins independent general practice in the United Kingdom within the context of the National Applied Health Service. Candidates who pass this assessment will have demonstrated their competence in applying knowledge at a level which is sufficiently high for independent practice.

Candidates may sit the AKT at any time during their training, but are advised by the RCGP that the paper is best taken while working in general practice as an ST3.

The exam takes the form of a three hour multiple-choice test of 200 single best answer, extended matching, algorithm completion, and picture questions. Other question formats include table completion and fill-in-the-blanks narratives. The question breakdown is approximately 80% clinical medicine, 10% critical appraisal/evidence-based clinical practice, and 10% health informatics and administrative issues.

The exam can currently be taken at one of three sittings a year in January, April and October, with the results released a month later. Candidates apply to sit the test online via the RCGP website (www.rcgp.org.uk) and then contact Pearson VUE to choose a test centre. There are around 150 centres throughout the UK so there is bound to be one nearby; however, the earlier a candidate books, the more likely their chances of sitting their exam at a venue of their choice.

The exam is computer-based, but a pen and wipe-clean board are provided for each candidate for rough work. Please note that candidates are not permitted to take anything (including food, drink, pens, paper or watches) into the test room and CCTV cameras are used to ensure there are no violations of test security.

I would highly recommend that candidates visit the Pearson VUE website (www.pearsonvue.com/rcgp) to familiarise themselves with the layout of a typical centre and take the tutorial in computer-based testing.

The good news, however, is that there are no limits to the number of attempts that can be made and approximately 80% of candidates pass. Also, there are no multiple true/false questions or negative marking so, if in doubt, make an educated guess!

Preparation

My main advice here would be to practise as many questions as you can – for those questions you get wrong, see this as an educational gap and try to fill it – and read around the subject using journals such as the *BJGP* and *BMJ*; other good sources of information are the *Drugs and Therapeutic Bulletin* and the *BNF*. Also, make use of the internet and visit sites such as NICE and SIGN; Bandolier is also useful. The sacred texts by Neighbour, Pendleton, Berne and Balint are not only helpful for the exam, they are also quite interesting.

You should use the questions in this book to guide your studying rather than trying to read everything ever written and then attempt the questions. Beware of concentrating your reading on subjects you already know well. As Confucius said:

> *If you know, recognize that you know,*
> *If you don't know, realize that you don't know,*
> *That is Knowledge.*

I would also suggest visiting the RCGP website which has a wealth of information on the exam including sample questions and feedback on past papers; if they have identified an area for concern in previous candidates' performance they *will* retest it.

Certain topics such as statistics, epidemiology, sick certification, mental health Sections, benefits and DVLA exclusions lend themselves to MCQ and so these should be known well. Candidates have often said they find practice management issues difficult to revise: I would suggest spending some time with all the members in the primary care team to understand what their roles are, but especially the practice manager: you can ask them to explain concepts such as risk management, employment law, etc. Make the most of your year in general practice and get involved in practice issues by attending practice meetings.

It is helpful to get together with a group of colleagues to go over question papers together, share ideas and support one another. You may well remember something you talked about better than something you read.

The exam is written by practising general practitioners and based on everyday practice – it helps to keep a diary of PUNS and DENS so that you can look up areas of weakness and make notes as you go along; this is also a good habit to get into for appraisal later on.

The night before the exam, relax with a warm bath; go to bed early and get a good night's sleep; for those of you with responsibilities such as small children, ask someone else to look after them for the night. Make sure you know where you are going and what time you need to be there: ideally do a practice run of your route beforehand and have a look at the building where you'll be tested: familiarity with the venue is always helpful. On the day of the exam avoid too many stimulants: you will be wired enough as it is and extra caffeine will only make you agitated and cause a diuresis.

Passing the exam is not just about knowledge base, but also exam technique. Familiarise yourselves with terms such as pathognomonic, diagnostic, frequently, significantly, characteristically. Make sure you read the instructions for each question carefully: look out for negatives (e.g. which one of the following is NOT a side-effect?) before clicking the mouse on the correct box; if you don't know the answer to a question or are getting bogged down, make an educated guess, as gut feeling is often right. Most importantly, keep an eye on the time – a timer on the screen will tell you how much you have left. At the end, check through your work and then walk away; post mortems are never helpful.

Best of luck!

Questions 1–50

for answers see pages 13–20

1. Dementia and driving

A 72 year old man presents with a five month history strongly suggestive of Alzheimer's disease having scored 22/30 on MMSE; this is confirmed by the local psychogeriatrician. You know that he is driving.

Which one of the following is true?
A   GP must inform the DVLA immediately
B   There is a very high risk of car crashes in drivers with dementia in the first few years of presentation
C   Licences are normally valid up to the age of 70 years
D   GP must decide if the patient is fit to drive
E   DVLA states patients with mild, early dementia must not drive

2. Faecal incontinence

Which one of the following is true?
A   Prevalence of faecal incontinence in the community is 15%
B   Rectal bleeding, unexplained changes in bowel habit and anaemia should be investigated routinely
C   Obstetric history may be relevant
D   Loperamide hydrochloride is the second line treatment of choice for faecal incontinence associated with loose stools, when appropriate investigations and treatment have failed to resolve loose stool

3. BNF symbols

Which one of the following is true?
A   The black inverted triangle identifies drugs that have been licensed within the past year
B   The black inverted triangle signifies drugs that are exempt from MHRA's Yellow Card scheme
C   The black inverted triangle denotes newly licensed drugs that are being intensively monitored by MHRA
D   The black triangle denotes drugs that are soon to be off patent and are therefore likely to become cheaper
E   The black triangle denotes those drugs that can be bought over the counter

4-8. Back pain

A   Mechanical low back pain
B   Symphysis pubis dysfunction
C   Osteoporotic vertebral fracture
D   Ankylosing spondylitis
E   Spinal claudication
F   Neoplasm
G   Lumbar disc prolapse with sciatic nerve entrapment

For each scenario depicted below, select the single most likely diagnosis from the list above. Each stem may be used once, more than once, or not at all.

4.   A 23 year old trainee chef presents with a 4 month history of back pain and stiffness; this is always worse in the mornings and as a result he is often late for work; investigations show a raised ESR and you recall seeing his father in the past for back problems and uveitis.

5.   A 33 year old primigravida in her 20th week of pregnancy presents with sacroiliac and hip pain; she reports difficulty getting in and out of her car and a grinding sensation in the pubic area.

6.   A 62 year old lady presents with a constant gnawing pain localised to her thoracic spine; she was treated 2 years ago for breast cancer and is found to have a raised ESR. She notes her clothes are becoming looser.

7.   You are called to the home of a slim 58 year old lady who is complaining of acute, severe back pain; she is very tender over the thoraco–lumbar junction but there is no bruising visible; pain is worse if she coughs, when it radiates around ribs and waist to front; she recalls tripping slightly on the rug as she reached for her cigarettes. You note she was a ballerina in her youth.

8.   A 38 year old primary school teacher was helping her husband lay a patio over the weekend; she awoke the following morning with acute pain over her lower back, made worse by moving; she took some rest and the pain has responded well to paracetamol and ibuprofen; she is wondering whether to go back to work.

9. Carpal tunnel syndrome

Which one of the following is not associated with carpal tunnel syndrome?
A   Myxoedema
B   Diabetes mellitus
C   Acromegaly
D   Rheumatoid arthritis
E   Diabetes insipidus
F   Pregnancy
G   Amyloidosis

10. Cystic fibrosis

Which one of the following is true?
A   1 in 50 adults in the UK carry the CF gene
B   CF is equally common in all races
C   Positive sweat test is diagnostic
D   Patients require additional vitamins B, C and E
E   Boys and girls grow up to be infertile
F   10% of adults develop glucose intolerance

11–14. Heavy menstrual bleeding

Where no structural or histological abnormality is suspected, or revealed on examination and investigation, *which of the following (one in each case) would be most appropriate for the patients described below?*

A   Progesterone intrauterine system
B   Combined oral contraceptive pill
C   Low dose oral progesterones during luteal phase of menstrual cycle
D   Non-steroidal anti-inflammatory drugs
E   Tranexamic acid
F   Hysterectomy
G   Dilatation and curettage

11. 27 year old housewife had uncomplicated delivery 8/12 ago but experiencing regular heavy periods with flooding and clots since six months; not planning more children for at least another 2 years.

12. 18 year old student in steady relationship finding heavy bleeding difficult to cope with and interfering with studies. Smokes cigarettes, 5–10/day.

13. Heavy painful periods in 25 year old secretary; not in a relationship at moment, no contraceptive requirements. Fhx thrombophilia.

14. 42 year old lady with heavy periods and needing to use double sanitary protection; doesn't want hormones but does want something effective to make her bleeding lighter.

15. Heavy menstrual bleeding

Which one of the following investigations is recommended when a woman first presents with the problem of heavy bleeding during menstruation?

A Full blood count
B Serum ferritin
C Thyroid function tests
D Hormone profile
E Quantitative assessment of menstrual blood flow
F Saline infusion sonography

16. The menopause

All of the following parameters rise following the menopause, except which one?

A Ferritin
B FSH
C ESR
D Bilirubin
E Estradiol

17. Temporary residents

Temporary residents are correctly defined as living in the practice area for which one of the following periods?

A Less than 24 hours
B More than 24 hours, less than 1 week
C More than 72 hours, less than 1 week
D More than 24 hours, less than 72 hours
E More than 24 hours, less than 3 months

18. Smoking cessation

The National Institute for Health and Care Excellence (NICE) has been asked by the Department of Health to develop public health guidance on the use of tobacco harm reduction approaches to smoking cessation.

Which one of the following is not currently licensed as a nicotine-containing product?

A Transdermal patches
B Gum
C Tablets / lozenges
D Nasal / mouth spray
E Inhalator
F Electronic cigarettes

19. The Caldicott Guardian

The Caldicott Guardian's role is best described in terms of which one of the following?:
A   Patient confidentiality
B   Communicable disease control
C   Personnel security
D   Patient complaints
E   Practice accounts

20. Colic

With regard to colic, which one of the following statements is true?:
A   Affects 60% of babies
B   Tends to occur most commonly in first born males
C   Research shows that babies with colic tend not to eat or gain as much weight as their peers
D   Symptoms always occur during the evening
E   Rare before 2–4 weeks and can last 3 months or more

21. Systemic lupus erythematosus

The following factors are known to make SLE active, except which one?
A   Sunshine
B   Pregnancy
C   Stress
D   Infection
E   Steroids
F   Isoniazid

22-25. Paediatric orthopaedics

A   Transient synovitis of the hip
B   Slipped upper femoral epiphysis
C   Septic arthritis
D   Perthes' disease

Match the following presentations with the single most appropriate diagnosis from the list above.

22. 2 year old boy was walking well from 18 months of age, but over past two weeks is refusing to weight-bear and is complaining of 'leg hurting' and wants to be carried all the time.

23. 7 year old boy attends with mum giving one month history of pain in both knees; limping.

24. 14 year old boy presenting with pain at rest in groin, both sides; shy, overweight; limited abduction and medial rotation on examination; leg appears shortened and externally rotated.

25. 4 year old boy presenting with pain in right hip; lying quietly and very still; reluctant to be examined, systemically unwell.

26-32. Ophthalmology

A   Amaurosis fugax
B   Hyperthyroidism
C   Retinal vein occlusion
D   Uveitis
E   Herpes zoster
F   Herpes simplex
G   Optic neuritis
H   Vitreous haemorrhage
I   Foreign body

Match the following presentations with the single most appropriate diagnosis from the list above. Each stem may be used once, more than once, or not at all.

26. A 56 year old businessman who smokes heavily attends worried because he noticed a brief loss of vision, like a curtain coming over his right eye, whilst driving this morning; sight has returned to normal by the time he sees you.

27. A 25 year old mature student who is being seen by one of your partners for chronic low back pain and morning stiffness attends with acute onset of pain affecting the left eye, photophobia, blurred vision and watering of the eye.

28. A 67 year old gentleman presents with a blistering rash affecting his right upper eyelid and part of his forehead; the rash was preceded by a painful tingling sensation.

29. A 56 year old gentleman, who is known to have mixed hyperlipidaemia, presents having experienced sudden loss of vision affecting the right eye; on fundoscopy, the fundus looks like a stormy sunset with haemorrhages and engorged veins.

30. A 32 year old baker presents with pain, photophobia, blurred vision and watering of the eyes; when stained with fluorescein and viewed through a blue light, you notice what looks like a linear branching pattern on the surface of the eye. There is no history of trauma.

31. A 60 year old lady with a 20 year history of diabetes attends with a sudden, painless loss of vision; despite repeated adjustments to the lenses of your ophthalmoscope, you are unable to visualise the retina.

32. A 24 year old lady attends complaining of a gradual loss of colour discrimination over the past few weeks; eye movements are uncomfortable; a few weeks previously she experienced problems with her speech; six months ago she had an episode of pins and needles affecting her forearm which settled spontaneously by the time she saw the doctor; she is a teacher in a primary school and under a lot of stress at the moment.

33. Neurology

A 40 year old lorry driver attends complaining of numbness and weakness affecting his lower limbs; this started a few days ago in his lower legs but is progressing upwards and he has difficulty coming upstairs to your surgery room; he smokes 5–10 cigarettes per day and drinks 3 units of alcohol per week. He was last seen at the surgery 3 weeks ago with a viral sore throat for which he was advised to take paracetamol. On examination, he has absent ankle and weak knee reflexes.

Which one of the following is the most likely diagnosis?
A   Acute idiopathic polyneuritis
B   Cauda equina syndrome
C   Vitamin B6 deficiency
D   Vitamin B12 deficiency
E   Hansen's disease

34. Neurology

You are called to the home of an elderly lady who has been found collapsed next to her bed by her carer; she opens her eyes only when you ask her to, and offers her arm when you ask to do her blood pressure; her speech consists of inappropriate words.

Her Glasgow Coma Scale score is:
A   Twelve
B   Thirteen
C   Fourteen
D   Fifteen
E   Sixteen

35. Erectile dysfunction

Treatment on the NHS is available for all patients with erectile dysfunction except which one of the following groups?
A   Those with diabetes mellitus
B   Those with multiple sclerosis
C   Those with Parkinson's disease
D   Those already receiving treatment prior to 14 September 2008
E   Those with a single gene neurological disease

36-39. Physical examination

A 34.7 – 37.3
B 35.5 – 37.5
C 35.8 – 38.0
D 36.6 – 38.0

For each of the places of measurement below, select the single most appropriate normal temperature range in degrees Celsius from the list above.

36. Ear

37. Mouth

38. Axilla

39. Rectum

40. Venlafaxine

Which one of the following statements regarding venlafaxine is correct?
A Is considered superior to cognitive behavioural therapy in the management of mild depression
B Is the treatment of choice in the management of depression in patients with recent myocardial infarction or unstable angina
C Requires baseline ECG in all patients before initiating treatment and during
D Is an SNRI

41-46. Urology

A   Diabetes mellitus
B   Renal calculus
C   Nephrotic syndrome
D   Acute pyelonephritis
E   Transitional cell carcinoma of bladder
F   Chronic renal failure
G   Munchausen syndrome
H   Diabetes insipidus
I   Cystitis

Match the following presentations with the single most appropriate diagnosis from the list above. Each stem may be used once, more than once, or not at all.

41. 15 year old boy attends with mum complaining of fever and rigors; examination reveals mild left loin tenderness; dips urine shows turbid urine, positive for nitrites and leukocyte esterase.

42. 20 year old girl attends with increased appetite, thirst over past few weeks; dip urine shows positive for ketones and glucose; specific gravity is 1.010. She thinks that her clothes feel looser.

43. 4 year old boy attends with mum who is worried that he seems very lethargic over past couple of weeks and now she has also noticed he is looking puffy around the eyes; urine is cloudy, frothy, negative to nitrites and blood but positive to protein+++.

44. 50 year old man requests home visit after a sleepless night with intermittent waves of excruciating lower abdominal pain; on examination he is writhing around the bed, finding it difficult to get comfortable. Urine is cloudy with blood+++; negative to leukocyte esterase, nitrites, protein; microscopic urinalysis shows wbc 2–5/hpf, rbc >100/hpf.

45. A 21 year old catering assistant attends having slipped on a wet floor at work and landed awkwardly on his side; he has brought a urine sample with him. The sample is clear, red and negative to blood, glucose, protein, leukocyte esterase.

46. 60 year old man attends complaining of mild dysuria and occasional hesitancy for past few weeks; he is otherwise well, takes no medication, drinks 14 units of alcohol per week and smokes 40 cigarettes/day. Urine is positive to blood++ and there is a trace of protein, trace of ketones; urine is sent for microscopy and results return showing wbc<2/hpf, rbc 10–30/hpf, occasional hyaline casts and presence of atypical uroepithelial cells.

47-50. Target INR

A   2.0 – 3.0
B   2.5 – 3.5
C   3.0 – 4.0

Which one of the INR ranges given above is appropriate for each of the following diagnoses? Each option may be used once, more than once, or not at all.

47. Antiphospholipid syndrome

48. First below knee vein thrombosis and no persistent risk factors

49. First proximal vein thrombosis and no persistent risk factors

50. First generation mechanical prosthetic heart valve

Answers to questions 1-50

1. Answer C is true.

There is a growing population of elderly drivers in this country and a clinical review in June 2007 highlighted this (Breen *et al. BMJ*, 2007; **334**: 1365-9). Many people with early dementia can drive safely and the risk of crashes remains low up to three years in a large proportion; however, it is important to reach a balance between independence and safety.

The DVLA (www.dft.gov.uk/dvla) *At A Glance Guide* (revised March 2013) states that "group 1 licences are normally valid up to age 70; there is no upper age limit but after age 70 renewal is necessary every 3 years; all licence applications require a medical self declaration by the patient." It is then the legal responsibility of the DVLA to decide whether someone is medically unfit to drive.

It is the responsibility of the licence holder to disclose any medical condition that may impair his/her ability to drive; the GP must therefore make the patient aware of this at the time of diagnosis; he should repeat the advice verbally and in writing as necessary, and in the event that the patient continues to drive despite being warned of the dangers, or the patient does not understand (e.g. dementia), the GP may choose to breach confidentiality and inform the DVLA directly, having advised the patient that this is what he intends to do.

In early dementia, when sufficient skills are retained and progression is slow, a licence may be issued subject to annual review; a formal driving assessment may be necessary. However, those with poor cognition, disorientation and lack of insight or judgement are almost certainly not fit to drive (page 30 in DVLA *At a Glance Guide*).

2. Answer C is true.

NICE (2007) suggest that prevalence in the community is nearer 1-10%.

Symptoms suggestive of a lower GI cancer that warrant urgent referral include:
- palpable intraluminal rectal mass on DRE
- rectal bleeding and change in bowel habit for >6/52 in someone >40 years
- rectal bleeding and/or change in bowel habit for 6 weeks in someone >60 years
- RLQ abdominal mass suggestive of large bowel involvement
- unexplained Fe deficiency anaemia

(*NICE Referral Guidelines for Suspected Cancer CG27*, June 2005).
Women who have recently given birth are at high risk of faecal incontinence, especially if they have had a significant obstetric injury.

Loperamide is an anti-motility drug that works on opioid receptors in the bowel, reducing peristalsis, and is the drug of first choice.

3. Answer C is true.

The black triangle symbol denotes drugs that are newly licensed and are being intensively monitored for reported adverse reactions by the Medicines and Healthcare Products Regulatory Agency; yellow cards may be used to report such reactions and can be found at the back of the *BNF*, but reactions may also be reported online and a new pilot scheme has been introduced to encourage self-reporting by patients, parents and carers.

There is no standard time for which products retain a black triangle; safety data are usually reviewed after two years.

4. Answer D is correct.

Ankylosing spondylitis is associated with HLA B27; early X-rays show widening of SI joints and marginal sclerosis; later, fusion of SI joints and vertebral squaring and fusion (a.k.a. bamboo spine).

5. Answer B is correct.

Symphysis pubis dysfunction – due to the effect of pregnancy hormones on pelvic joints leading to inequalities in movement – sometimes causes quite disabling pain anywhere around the pelvic girdle; treatment is supportive with rest, painkillers, physiotherapy; usually resolves after delivery, may recur with subsequent births.

6. Answer F is correct.

Presentation of back pain in anyone under 20, or over 55, that has a constant, progressive, non-mechanical nature, and where there is a past history of cancer, is one of the so-called red flags for potentially serious spinal pathology and warrants urgent (<4/52) referral.

Other red flags are:
- history of HIV, systemic steroid, drug abuse
- systemically unwell, weight loss
- violent trauma
- thoracic pain, widespread neurology

7. Answer C is correct.

Other risk factors for osteoporotic fractures include systemic steroid use, family history of osteoporosis; encourage patients at risk to eat well and maintain BMI >19 kg m^{-2}, to take regular weight-bearing exercise, stop smoking, and take alcohol only within set limits; calcium and vitamin D supplements may be beneficial.

8. Answer A is correct.

The average GP sees >50 acute backs per year; 15 million work days are lost each year due to mechanical low back pain; most resolve within a few weeks; simple analgesia and early mobilisation are recommended in most patients.

9. Answer E is correct.

An easy way to remember the causes of carpal tunnel syndrome is: MEDIAN TRAP

Myxoedema
o**E**dema
Diabetes mellitus
Idiopathic
Acromegaly
Neoplastic

Trauma
Rheumatoid arthritis
Amyloidosis
Pregnancy

10. Answer C is correct.

1 in 25 adults in the UK carry the CF gene which is inherited in an autosomal recessive manner; it is most common in Caucasians, and rare in people of Afro-Caribbean origin. If both parents are carriers, there is a 1 in 4 chance of their offspring being affected.

There is a single gene mutation resulting in abnormal function of the CF conductance regulator; this is essential for trans cell membrane salt and water movement, resulting in thickened, salty secretions in the lung, gut and reproductive organs. Consequently, boys are azoospermic and infertile; girls, however, grow up to be sub-fertile and conception is possible.

Patients require pre-meal oral pancreatic enzymes (Creon), a high calorie diet, and supplements of fat-soluble vitamins A, D, and E.

The risk of impaired glucose tolerance is significant; the cumulative incidence of diabetes mellitus in a study in Denmark was 24% in patients aged 20, increasing to 76% in those age 30 (Lanng *et al. BMJ*, 1995; **311**: 655–9).

11. Answer A is correct.

LNG-IUS (Mirena) is suggested as the first-line treatment to be offered provided long-term use (>12/12) is anticipated; it is very effective and decreases blood loss by 90% when used over 12 months.

12. Answer B is correct.

Oral progestogens during the luteal phase are used by some GPs but are not recommended as they are not very effective when given at the usual low dose; they are considered third-line after COCP and non-hormonal methods (they can be used at higher doses of 5 mg t.d.s. starting 3 days before expected date of menstruation to postpone bleeding, but that is a different clinical scenario).

13. Answer D is correct.

NICE Clinical Guideline on Heavy Menstrual Bleeding (*CG44*, January 2007) states that when HMB coexists with dysmenorrhoea, NSAIDs should be preferred to tranexamic acid.

14. Answer E is correct.

Tranexamic acid is an anti-fibrinolytic agent and can reduce blood flow by 50%. Mefanamic acid (Ponstan) reduces bleeding by only 25–30% but is better for those with dysmenorrhoea. The other options are hormonal in nature; surgery would not be offered first-line.

> Note that D&C is an investigation, not a treatment!

15. Answer is A.

NICE Guidance (*CG44*, 2007, *Heavy menstrual bleeding*) does not recommend investigations other than FBC.

16. Answer is E.

ESR rises with increasing age.

17. Answer is E.

Anyone in the practice area for <24 hours, treated as an emergency or immediately requiring treatment; anyone residing for more than 24 hours and less than 3 months, as a temporary resident.

18. Answer is F.

Electronic cigarettes are battery-operated devices; they are not currently regulated by the Medicines and Healthcare Products Regulatory Agency, so are not licensed as a medicine in the UK.

The BMA (Jan 2013) has advised health professionals to use regulated and licensed nicotine replacement therapy to help patients stop smoking.

19. Answer is A.

The Caldicott Report was issued in December 1997 to help deal with concerns about the way patient information is used in the NHS, and due to concerns about confidentiality.

A senior health person should be nominated as 'the Guardian' in each health organisation and it is their remit to be responsible for safeguarding the confidentiality of patient-identifiable information, e.g. by using NHS number rather than name of patient wherever possible.

20. Answer is E.

Colic is diagnosed when there is uncontrolled, extended crying in an otherwise healthy baby for longer than three hours every day for more than three days in a week; it is the extreme end of normal crying behaviour; harmless, but can be distressing for carers.

Affects 20% of babies; m=f; it is pyloric stenosis that is classically seen in first born males!

Cause unknown, no proven treatment, but research shows that babies with colic continue to eat and gain weight normally. No medical treatment needed or proven, but do take a full history, undertake a thorough examination, and be supportive to parents.

Colic can cause much stress to unsupported individuals with poor coping strategies and the child may be at risk of abuse: helpful contacts: Cry-sis (www.cry-sis.org.uk) and National Childbirth Trust (www.nct.org.uk).

21. Answer is E.

SLE is a rare autoimmune disease with variable presentation and multi-system involvement: arthritis, photo sensitivity, butterfly facial rash, fibrosing alveolitis, pneumonitis, glomerulonephritis, pericarditis, cranial nerve lesions and anaemia being just some of its myriad presentations. 95% of patients are ANA (anti-nuclear antibody positive) on autoimmune profile testing.

An easy way to remember activators is UV PRISM:

UV – sunlight

Pregnancy
Reducing steroids
Infection – viral, bacterial
Stress
More drugs

Steroids are the mainstay of treatment; isoniazid, procainamide, hydralazine and some antibiotics have been implicated in drug-induced SLE.

22. Answer is A.
Also known as irritable hip – cause unknown; peak age 2–10 years; m>f; exclude septic arthritis; usually resolves spontaneously after 1–2 weeks.

23. Answer is D.
Perthes' disease – due to avascular necrosis of the femoral head; bilateral in 10%; peak age 4–7 years; m>f. Refer to orthopaedics for X-ray, rest, bracing, +/– surgery.

24. Answer is B.
SUFE – typically overweight underdeveloped children, or tall thin boys, aged 10–15 years; m>f; X-rays show backwards and downwards slip of femoral epiphysis with respect to femoral head; refer to orthopaedics for surgical pinning / reconstructive surgery.

25. Answer is C.
Septic arthritis of any joint is an emergency – child is very unwell; needs to be admitted for i.v. antibiotics.

26. Answer is A.

Amaurosis fugax is caused by retinal emboli from ipsilateral carotid disease causing a temporary interruption to retinal circulation.

27. Answer is D.

The cause of the mature student's back pain and stiffness was ankylosing spondylitis, a common association of which is anterior uveitis.

28. Answer is E.

Herpes zoster ophthalmicus involves the tissues innervated by the ophthalmic division of the trigeminal nerve and accounts for 10–25% of all cases of shingles.

29. Answer is C.

Retinal vein occlusion can be of a branch or a central vein; as well as hyperlipidaemia, it is also associated with hypertension and hyperviscosity.

30. Answer is F.

Fluorescein staining of a dendritic ulcer caused by herpes simplex will show up when viewed through a blue light – treatment is with acyclovir eye drops – never use steroids as massive amoeboid ulceration and blindness can result.

31. Answer is H.

The painless loss of vision may be preceded by a storm of red floaters; one is unable to visualise the retina because of the haemorrhage within the orbit.

32. Answer is G.

Optic neuritis can be a presenting symptom of multiple sclerosis.

33. Answer is A.

Also known as Guillain–Barré syndrome. Hansen's disease is leprosy.

34. Answer is A.

Based on the Glasgow Coma Scale (see below), her best eye opening response is 3, her best verbal response is 3 and her best motor response is six. Please note that the maximum possible GCS score a patient can have is 15.

	1	2	3	4	5	6
Eyes	Does not open eyes	Opens eyes in response to painful stimuli	Opens eyes in response to voice	Opens eyes spontaneously	N/A	N/A
Verbal	Makes no sounds	Incomprehensible sounds	Utters inappropriate words	Confused, disoriented	Oriented, converses normally	N/A
Motor	Makes no movements	Extension to painful stimuli	Abnormal flexion to painful stimuli	Flexion / withdrawal to painful stimuli	Localises painful stimuli	Obeys commands

35. Answer is D.

The correct date is 14/9/1998 (*BNF 58*, Sept 2009).

Questions 36–39: All answers taken from *Oxford Handbook of General Practice* (2009)

36. Answer is C.

Normal ear temperature ranges from 35.8 to 38.0°C.

37. Answer is B.

Normal oral temperature range is 35.5 to 37.5°C.

38. Answer is A.

Normal axillary temperature is 34.7 to 37.3°C.

39. Answer is D.

Normal rectal temperature is 36.6 to 38.0°C.

40. Answer D is true.

CBT and self help should be considered first-line in management of mild depression, rather than antidepressants because the risk-benefit ratio is low; if an antidepressant is to be prescribed, current guidance states that an SSRI is normally chosen, bearing in mind an association with increased risk of bleeding and drug interactions. For people who have a chronic physical health problem, consider using citalopram or sertraline, because these have a lower propensity for interactions.

Regarding venlafaxine, this should *not* be prescribed to those who have had a recent MI, are at risk of arrhythmias, or have uncontrolled hypertension. Also, take into account toxicity in overdose for people at significant risk of suicide and be aware that, compared with other equally effective antidepressants recommended in primary care, venlafaxine is associated with a greater risk of death from overdose; the greatest risk in overdose is with tricyclic antidepressants (TCAs), except for lofepramine.

NICE Guidance CG90 (October 2009) *Depression: treatment and management of depression in adults, including adults with a chronic physical health problem.*

41. Answer is D.

Turbid urine, fever, tenderness and a dipstick positive for leukocyte esterase all point to infection; loin pain and being acutely unwell suggest pyelonephritis.

42. Answer is A.

Positive glucose indicates diabetes; positive ketones indicate insulin is lacking and that adipose tissue is being metabolised, typical of IDDM; in the absence of glucosuria, ketone bodies suggest starvation.

43. Answer is C.

The loosest skin in a child is peri-orbital, so this is the first place that oedema is often noticed; the most common cause of nephrotic syndrome in children is minimal change glomerulonephritis.

44. Answer is B.

Haematuria can be due to numerous causes including inflammation, trauma, glomerulonephritis, calculi, instrumentation, neoplasms, etc; however, the severe pain suggests calculus.

45. Answer is G.

The macroscopic appearance would suggest haematuria, but the dipstick for blood is negative; this could be as a result of food colouring.

46. Answer is E.

Haematuria with atypical uroepithelial cells in a heavy smoker should prompt an urgent referral to urologists (2 week rule); smoking, exposure to beta-naphthylamine and analine dyes (rubber, petrochemical, paint, textile, petroleum industries) are also risk factors.

47. Answer is A.

Baglin *et al.* (*British Journal of Haematology*, 2006; **132**: 227–85) quote two randomised trials comparing a target INR of 2.5 (range 2.0–3.0) to a target greater than 3.0 (3.1–4.0); based on these studies, both groups of authors (Crowther *et al.* 2003; and Finazzi *et al.* 2005), concluded that a target INR of 2.5 was sufficient for the treatment of patients with thrombosis (venous or arterial) in association with anti-phospholipid syndrome; there are insufficient data to make an evidence-based recommendation for patients with anti-phospholipid syndrome and arterial thrombosis, but a higher target of 3.5 is often used.

48. Answer is A.

Target INR is 2.5 – grade A recommendation as per Baglin *et al.* (*British Journal of Haematology*, 2006; **132**: 227–85).

49. Answer is A.

Target INR is 2.5 – grade A recommendation as per Baglin *et al.* (*British Journal of Haematology*, 2006; **132**: 227–85).

50. Answer is C.

The newer second generation heart valves have a target INR of 3.0 (2.5–3.5) .

Questions 51–100

for answers see pages 31–37

51. Abdominal pain

Abdominal pain in a 4 year old can be the presenting feature of all the following except which one?

A Viral infection
B Appendicitis
C Meningitis
D Pneumonia
E Hypertrophic pyloric stenosis
F Migraine

52–55. Leg ulcers

A Neuropathic
B Arterial
C Neoplastic
D Venous

Match the possible leg ulcer diagnoses to the scenarios below. Each answer can be used only once.

52. A 75 year old Caucasian lady presents with an 18 month history of a shallow, intermittently healing leg ulcer, situated above the left medial malleolus. There is marked bilateral peripheral oedema.

53. An 80 year old man, known to be hypertensive and a heavy smoker, presents with a painful lesion at the tip of his left toe; he has been complaining of calf pain when he walks. The ulcer has a punched out appearance to it.

54. An obese 76 year old diabetic Asian lady attends with her son who is concerned about a foot infection; on examination, there is a deep painless ulcer over the head of the metatarsal of her left foot.

55. A 67 year old man with a long-standing venous ulcer has been seeing the practice nurse for treatment; she is concerned because the edge of the ulcer is not healing and the edges have started to evert.

56-66. Drug side-effects

A Glyceryl trinitrate
B Thyroxine
C Methotrexate
D Zopiclone
E Mesalazine
F Enalapril
G Micronor
H Rifampicin
I Atenolol
J Bendrofluazide
K Prednisolone
L Heparin
M Finasteride
N Eflornithine
O Oxytetracycline

Match the side-effects below to the drug most likely to cause them from the list above; match only one drug to each side-effect; not all the drugs will be matched. Note: there is more than one possible answer to some of the questions.

56. Adrenal suppression

57. Headache

58. Haemopoietic suppression

59. Gout

60. Exacerbation of Raynaud's phenomenon

61. Metallic taste in mouth

62. Dry cough

63. Orange-red tears

64. Hair growth

65. Hair loss

66. Staining of growing bones and teeth

67. Adiposity

Which one of the following is the most generally accepted measure of general adiposity in adults?

A Body Mass Index (BMI) centile
B Waist to hip ratio
C BMI
D Bioimpedance
E BMI z-score

68. Bariatric surgery

Which one of the following is not a mandatory criterion for referring an adult for bariatric surgery?

A The person commits to the need for long-term follow-up
B The person has received or will be receiving intensive management in a specialist obesity service
C The person has a BMI of 40 kg/m² or more, or between 35 kg/m² and 40kg/m² and other significant disease (for example, type 2 diabetes or high blood pressure) that could be improved if they lost weight
D The person is generally fit for anaesthesia or surgery
E All appropriate non-surgical measures have been tried but have failed to achieve or maintain adequate, clinically beneficial weight loss for at least 12 months

69. Physical activity

What are the current levels of physical activity recommended by the Chief Medical Officer (CMO) for adults (i.e. those aged 19-64) to achieve general health benefit? Choose only one answer.

A 150 minutes of moderate intensity aerobic activity such as cycling or fast walking every week
B 150 minutes of moderate intensity aerobic activity such as cycling or fast walking every week or muscle strengthening activities on two or more days a week that work all major muscle groups
C 150 minutes of moderate intensity aerobic activity such as cycling or fast walking every week as well as muscle strengthening activities on two or more days a week that work all major muscle groups
D 60 minutes of vigorous intensity aerobic activity such as running or singles tennis every week and muscle strengthening activities on two or more days a week that work all major muscle groups

70-72. Anaemia

Given normal values as follows:
- Hb 13.0–17.0 g/l (male)
- WCC 4.0–11.0 × 10^9/l
- platelets 150–400 × 10^9/l
- MCV 80–100 fl

A   Iron deficiency
B   Alcoholic liver disease
C   Aplastic anaemia
D   Sickle cell anaemia
E   Autoimmune haemolytic anaemia

For each of the results below, select the single most likely diagnosis from the list of options above.

70. Hb 8.2, WCC 6.3, platelets 246, MCV 110

71. Hb 5.1, WCC 0.4, platelets 34, MCV 84

72. Hb 9.4, WCC 7.9, platelets 175, MCV 76

73. Breast cancer

Risk factors for breast cancer include all except which one of the following?:

A   High saturated fat intake
B   Unopposed oestrogen therapy
C   Breast feeding
D   Early menarche
E   Nulliparity

74. Feverish illness in children

Which one of the following is untrue?

A   Oral routes may be routinely used to measure the body temperature of children aged 0–5 years

B   In infants under the age of 4 weeks, body temperature should be measured with an electronic thermometer in the axilla

C   In children aged 4 weeks to 5 years, body temperature may be measured by either an electronic thermometer in the axilla, chemical dot thermometer in the axilla or infra-red tympanic thermometer

D   A capillary refill time of 3 seconds or longer is an immediate-risk group marker for serious illness ('red' sign)

E   Reported parental perception of a fever is considered valid and should be taken seriously by healthcare professionals

75–79. Chest pain

A   Myocardial infarction
B   Pleurisy
C   Hyperventilation
D   Pneumothorax
E   Herpes zoster
F   Herpes simplex
G   Post-herpetic neuralgia
H   Fractured rib

Match one diagnosis above to each scenario below.

75. An 18 year old lady presents with difficulty breathing, chest tightness, and perioral paraesthesia; her heart sounds, breath sounds, bp and peak flow are all normal; she is tachypnoeic and is gasping for breath.

76. A 58 year old hypertensive man presents with sudden onset crushing central chest pain radiating to the jaw and left shoulder; he is pale, sweaty and vomits once.

77. A tall slim 21 year old male presents with sudden onset left-sided chest pain; he is dyspnoeic; the percussion note is resonant and breath sounds are reduced on the left; the trachea has been pushed over to the right.

78. A 78 year old lady in a nursing home presents with pain over the right side of her chest; she was seen by your colleague 2 days previously who thought the pain was musculoskeletal in origin; on examination she has a very painful vesicular rash affecting the T8 dermatome.

79. The previous lady is seen again a few weeks later; the rash has disappeared but the area remains exquisitely sensitive.

80. Immunisation schedule

Tom is a healthy newborn who attends for his six week check; mum is very keen to discuss which immunisations he will be having.

At which one of the following appointments will Tom not be receiving a dose of PCV (pneumococcal conjugate vaccine)?

A Two months
B Three months
C Four months
D Thirteen months

81-85. Antibiotic treatment

A Flucloxacillin
B Penicillin V
C Co-amoxiclav
D Benzylpenicillin
E Amoxicillin
F Methicillin
G Penicillin and flucloxacillin
H None of these

Match the scenarios given below to the single most appropriate antibiotic treatment; each response may be used once, more than once or not at all.

81. A school teacher attends having been bitten the previous day by the class pet hamster; she has a small bite on the back of the left hand which looks inflamed; she is otherwise well.

82. A 1 year old child with headache, dislike of bright light and leg pains; on examination he has neck stiffness and a petechial rash.

83. A 15 year old girl complaining of a sore throat, fatigue and pyrexia for 10 days; examination shows sore throat, enlarged cervical and occipital lymph nodes; positive monospot blood test result received from lab.

84. A 37 year old checkout assistant presents with fever, malaise, cough productive of purulent sputum and right-sided pleuritic chest pain; coarse crackles can be heard at the right side of the chest.

85. A 4 year old child with red patch on cheek, covered in a golden crust. Child is otherwise well.

86-87. Genetics

A   HLA DR2
B   HLA DR3
C   HLA DR4

Match the disease to the genetic marker; there is only one correct answer; each response may be used once, more than once or not at all.

86. Addison's disease

87. Graves' disease

88. Sports medicine – banned substances

All of the following substances are banned in sports except which one?

A   anabolic steroids
B   human growth hormone
C   heroin
D   amphetamines
E   caffeine
F   diuretics

89-90. Classes of illegal drugs

A   Class A
B   Class B
C   Class C

Match the class to the drugs below (based on the Misuse of Drugs Act 1971).

89. Cannabis.

90. Cocaine, LSD.

91. LARC: Depo

Considering long-acting contraception in the form of Depo Provera, which one of the following statements is true?

A Depo should automatically be used as first-line contraception for adolescents and teenagers
B Depo may be used in women with risk factors for osteoporosis
C Depo causes a reduction in BMI in most women
D In women of all ages, one should carefully evaluate the pros and cons if the woman plans to use Depo for more than 2 years

92-98. Sick certification

A Med 3 statement of fitness to work
B Med 4
C Med 5
D Med 6
E MatB1
F RM7
G DS1500 report
H SC1
I SC2
J Med 10

Match one certificate to each situation below. Each option may be used once, more than once or not at all.

92. You are in doubt regarding the incapacity of the patient.

93. Your patient is receiving antiviral treatment for HIV which is making them feel very nauseous; they are worried that entering an exact diagnosis may cause significant discrimination towards them at work.

94. Your patient was recently in hospital for tooth extraction. He has been given a form by the nursing sister on the ward to confirm he was in hospital as an inpatient.

95. Mum-to-be in 21st week of pregnancy requires a certificate to allow her to claim statutory maternity pay.

96. Family attend requesting medical certificate – father is terminally ill and likely to die within 6 months.

97. First seven days of illness for self-employed plumber; not entitled to statutory sick pay.

98. First seven days of illness for employee of plumber; entitled to statutory sick pay.

99. Irritable bowel syndrome

Which one of the following list is not one of the Manning Criteria for diagnosis of IBS?

A   Abdominal pain
B   Increased stool frequency with pain
C   Looser stool with pain
D   Feeling of incomplete evacuation
E   Mucus in stool
F   Blood in stool
G   Relief of pain with defecation

100. Back pain

Which one of the following statements regarding the management of acute back pain is false?

A   NSAIDs are no better than placebo for acute pain
B   Muscle relaxants relieve pain more than placebo
C   There is strong evidence to suggest that bed-rest and specific exercises are not effective
D   Spinal manipulation may be considered for pain relief
E   Concordance with advice to stay active decreases chronic disability

Answers to questions 51–100

51. Answer E is untrue.
Abdominal pain in a four year old can be due to a dozen different reasons, not all of them intra-abdominal! Pyloric stenosis, however, presents with projectile vomiting, typically around the sixth week of life.

52. Answer is D.
Venous ulcers (which account for 70% of leg ulcers) are associated with a history of DVT, obesity, varicose veins, smoking; they have a shallow sloping edge and are often surrounded by an area of lipodermatosclerosis and varicose eczema; patients should have an ankle brachial pressure index done and if this is >0.8 and there are no contraindications, multi-layered, elastic, high compression bandaging should be applied.

53. Answer is B.
Arterial ulcers (which account for 10% of leg ulcers) are more painful when the legs are elevated but gravity helps increase blood flow when legs are dependent with consequent dependent rubor; unlike venous ulcers, they are usually dry. Associated gangrenous toes may be seen.

54. Answer is A.
Diabetic patients are at increased risk of arterial ulcers; however, their sensory perception is impaired because of neuropathy and so they are at risk of pressure from ill-fitting shoes – hence need for foot check as part of diabetes review in general practice.

55. Answer is C.
SIGN Guidelines (1998) state that if an ulcer is not healing after 12/52 or is showing suspicious changes such as a raised, rolled or everted edge, the patient should be referred for biopsy as the ulcer may be undergoing malignant change (Marjolin's ulcer). Also look at *NICE CG10 – Type 2 diabetes: Prevention and management of foot problems* (Jan 2004).

Questions 56–59: All answers taken from *BNF 58* (September 2009)

56. Answer is K.
Long-term steroids can also cause cataracts and osteoporosis.

57. Answer is A, but E is also a possibility (though less likely).
Headache caused by GTN tablet can be alleviated by swallowing tablet as stomach acids will inactivate it – this is why it needs to be taken sub-lingually, not orally.

58. Answer is C, but E is also a possibility (though less likely)

Patients need to have FBC, U/E and LFT before treatment, weekly for six months and then every 2–3 months; patients are advised not to self-medicate with aspirin or ibuprofen; alcohol should be avoided; all symptoms/signs of infection (especially sore throat) should be reported immediately.

59. Answer is J.

Thiazides can cause hyperuricaemia and gout.

60. Answer is I.

Beta blockers are contraindicated in severe peripheral vascular disease.

61. Answer is D.

Taste disturbance is associated with metronidazole, amiodarone, sulphasalazine, metformin and zopiclone – the last two typically leaving a metallic taste in the mouth.

62. Answer is F.

ACE inhibitors inhibit the breakdown of bradykinin and other kinins; angiotensin–II receptor antagonists, however, do not and so may be prescribed in those for whom the cough is troublesome.

63. Answer is H.

Urine, saliva and other body secretions are coloured orange–red by rifampicin and, unless warned, patients may be alarmed.

64. Answer is M, but G is also a possibility (though less likely).

Finasteride as 5 mg daily is prescribable on the NHS for BPH; as a treatment for male pattern baldness (1 mg o.d.) it is not available on the NHS.

65. Answer is N, but E and F are also possibilities (though less likely).

Eflornithine (Vaniqa) is a topical agent used to treat facial hirsutism in women; the two agents currently available to treat hair loss are finasteride in men and minoxidil in men and women.

66. Answer is O.

Deposition of tetracyclines in growing bones and teeth causes staining and occasionally dental hypoplasia; they should not be given to children under 12 or to pregnant/breast-feeding women.

67. Answer C is true.

According to *NICE guidance on the prevention, identification, assessment and management of overweight and obesity in adults and children* (*CG43*, December 2006), BMI is the most widely accepted measure of *general* adiposity in the adult population. Adults with a BMI of 25 kg/m² are defined as overweight and those with a BMI of over 30 kg/m² are defined as obese.

Waist circumference is a useful measure of *central* adiposity in adults. Men with a waist circumference of 94 cm or more are at increased risk of health problems. If their waist circumference is 102 cm or more, even at a healthy weight (BMI 18.5–25 kg/m²) they are at increased risk. Women with a waist circumference of 80 cm or more are at increased risk of health problems. If their waist circumference is 88 cm or more, even at a healthy weight (BMI 18.5–25 kg/m²) they are at increased risk.

Waist-to-hip ratio is a useful measure of central adiposity in adults, but is more difficult to measure. There is no evidence on the utility of bioimpedance compared with BMI in adults.

BMI centile cut-offs are used as a measure of adiposity and adiposity change in children.

68. Answer E is untrue.

The time period for achieving or maintaining adequate, clinically beneficial weight loss prior to referral for surgery is 6 months. However, all the other criteria must be fulfilled.

Bariatric surgery is also recommended as a first-line option (instead of lifestyle interventions or drug treatment) for adults with a BMI of more than 50 kg/m² in whom surgical intervention is considered appropriate. Surgery for obesity should only be undertaken by a multidisciplinary team after a comprehensive preoperative assessment of any psychological or clinical factors that may affect adherence to post-operative requirements. See *NICE CG43*, Dec 2006, *Obesity*.

69. Answer C is true.

The chief medical officer reviewed previously issued guidelines in 2011; the new guidelines are based on a comprehensive review of the latest evidence on physical activity and health and are now much more in line with those used in the USA. As well as aerobic activity, recommendations have been made for muscle building and bone strengthening activities such as lifting weights and yoga (www.gov.uk/government/publications/uk-physical-activity-guidelines [accessed 1 July 2013]).

70. Answer is B, but E is also a possibility (though less likely).

Macrocytic anaemias are also found in hypothyroidism. Could also be E if there was a marked reticulocytosis pushing up the MCV.

71. Answer is C.

All parameters are low, this is aplastic anaemia.

72. Answer is A.

Iron deficiency presents as a hypochromic, microcytic picture.

73. Answer C is untrue.

Breast cancer is the commonest cause of cancer deaths in women, accounting for 18% of all female cancer deaths; British women have a 1:9 lifetime risk of developing this disease.

It increases with age; risk factors include nulliparity, early menarche, late menopause, oestrogen therapy unopposed by progesterone, positive family history and saturated fat intake; early first child and breast-feeding are protective.

74. Answer A is untrue.

NICE advises that one should not routinely use the oral and rectal routes to measure the body temperature of children aged 0–5 years (*NICE CG160*, May 2013, *Feverish illness in children: Assessment and initial management in children younger than 5 years*. This guideline updates and replaces *NICE CG47, Feverish illness in children*.)

75. Answer is C.

76. Answer is A.

77. Answer is D.

78. Answer is E.

79. Answer is G

80. Answer is B.

When to immunise	Diseases protected against	Vaccine given
Two months old	Diphtheria, tetanus, pertussis (whooping cough), polio and *Haemophilus influenzae* type b (Hib) Pneumococcal infection	DTaP/IPV/Hib + Pneumococcal conjugate vaccine (PCV)
Three months old	Diphtheria, tetanus, pertussis, polio and *Haemophilus influenzae* type b (Hib) Meningitis C	DTaP/IPV/Hib + MenC
Four months old	Diphtheria, tetanus, pertussis, polio and *Haemophilus influenzae* type b (Hib) Meningitis C Pneumococcal infection	DTaP/IPV/Hib + MenC + PCV
Around 12 months	*Haemophilus influenzae* type b (Hib) Meningitis C	Hib/MenC
Around 13 months old	Measles, mumps and rubella Pneumococcal infection	MMR + PCV
Three years and four months or soon after	Diphtheria, tetanus, pertussis and polio Measles, mumps and rubella	DTaP/IPV or dTaP/IPV +MMR
Girls aged 12 to 13 years	Cervical cancer caused by human papillomavirus types 16 and 18	HPV
13 to 18 years old	Diphtheria, tetanus, polio	Td/IPV

Note: Tuberculosis and hepatitis B are non-routine immunisations for at-risk babies.

From July 2013, rotavirus will join the immunisation schedule as an oral two-dose vaccine given at the same time as other routine vaccines by the age of four months (www.gov.uk/government/organisations/public-health-england/series/rotavirus-vaccination-progarmme-for-infants [accessed 1 July 2013]).

81. Answer is C.

Co-amoxiclav is suggested by *BNF* for animal bites.

82. Answer is D.

Pre-hospital administration of benzylpenicillin has been recommended since 1988, and expert guidelines continue to recommend that all GPs carry it and inject it unless there is a history of immediate allergic reactions after previous penicillin administration. In this situation third-generation cephalosporins (cefotaxime rather than ceftriaxone for first-line use in meningococcal septicaemia) and chloramphenicol are recommended alternatives if available (*Meningococcal Meningitis and Septicaemia Guidance Notes*, Meningitis Research Foundation, 2008).

Do not give antibiotics, however, if this will delay urgent transfer to hospital (*NICE CG102*, June 2010, *The management of bacterial meningitis and meningococcal septicaemia in children and young people younger than 16 years in primary and secondary care*).

83. Answer is H.

None of the above as the girl has glandular fever; in particular, she should not be given amoxicillin which can cause a rash. Symptomatic treatment is advised.

84. Answer is E.

Amoxicillin, because this is a community-acquired pneumonia.

85. Answer is A.

Flucloxacillin for impetigo.

86. Answer is B.

87. Answer is B.

Addison's disease and Graves' disease are both associated with HLA DR3. HLA DR4 is associated with rheumatoid arthritis. HLA DR2 may be associated with osteoarthritis and with multiple sclerosis.

88. Answer is E.

Caffeine is allowed within permitted blood levels. Diuretics are useful to maintain fighting weight; frusemide can be used as a masking agent of other drugs in the urine.

Various drugs used to treat medical conditions, e.g. steroids, beta blockers, insulin, clomiphene, and tamoxifen, are also subject to restrictions; in such cases, the athlete has to submit a TUE (therapeutic use exemption form) and prove that they have the medical condition mentioned *and* that they need to take medication for it.

Cold/cough remedies include banned stimulants such as ephedrine and pseudo-ephedrine.

The only medications known to be OK are paracetamol and ibuprofen.

89. Answer is B.

Cannabis was reupgraded from Class C to Class B in 2009.

90. Answer is A.

Heroin, methadone and ecstasy are all Class A drugs.

91. Answer D is true.

It is known that DMPA can reduce bone mineral density (BMD) and recent studies have confirmed this; the CSM therefore issued a warning to this effect in Nov 2004 (www.mhra.gov.uk); the reduction in BMD is constant, then plateaus after a few years; it is not known to what extent the BMD recovers, and this may be particularly important in adolescents who have yet to reach full bone mass; for this reason, although Depo can be used, it should only be used when other methods are unacceptable or unsuitable.

92. Answer is A.

93. Answer is A.

94. Answer is J.

95. Answer is E.

96. Answer is G.

97. Answer is H.

98. Answer is I.

On 6 April 2010, the current Forms Med 3 and Med 5 were replaced with a single revised Statement of Fitness for Work.

In addition, forms RM7, Med 4 and MED 6 were withdrawn from use.

Originally, form RM7 allowed certifying doctors to request an independent medical assessment of their patient if the patient was making a claim to benefit; the Med 6 allowed certifying doctors to inform the Department for Work and Pensions that a less precise diagnosis had been completed on a Statement.

If, with the current forms, you feel making an accurate diagnosis would be harmful to your patient's wellbeing or compromise their position with their employer (for example because it would cause significant discrimination to them in the workplace), then it is acceptable to agree with your patient to enter a less precise diagnosis on the Med 3.

The original RM7 forms are no longer necessary because the majority of patients making a new claim to Employment and Support Allowance undergo a medical assessment within a short period of time after making the claim to benefit. (www.gov.uk/government/organisations/department-for-work-pensions/series/fit-note [accessed 1 July 2013])

99. Answer is F.

All of the others are in the Manning list of criteria, where if three or more are present, and there are no red flags, then a positive diagnosis of IBS can be made; blood in stool, weight loss, fever, anaemia or new symptoms in anyone over the age of 50 are all red flags and a full GI work-up is needed (*BMJ*, 2005; **330**: 632).

However, a recent systematic review and meta-analysis of observational studies, all of which were conducted in secondary care, showed that these criteria have not been validated extensively, and do not predict IBS with any great accuracy. In primary care most GPs benefit from using a symptom-based approach (*BMJ*, 2012; **345**: e5836).

In addition, NICE have clarified the situation further in *CG61* (*Irritable bowel syndrome in adults: diagnosis and management of irritable bowel syndrome in primary care*, February 2008).

100. Answer A is false.

NSAIDs are better than placebo for acute back pain; the *BMJ* (2006; **332**: 1430) states that regular paracetamol and NSAIDs should be used; NICE suggest paracetamol should be offered first-line, but when regular paracetamol alone is insufficient (and taking account of individual risk of side-effects and patient preference), NSAIDs and/or weak opioids may be used (*CG88, Low back pain: early management of persistent non-specific low back pain*, May 2009). Muscle relaxants and short-term opioids may be considered, and also spinal manipulation.

Questions 101–150

for answers see pages 49–57

101. Secondary diabetes mellitus

The following are all associated with secondary diabetes mellitus, except which one?
A   Thiazide diuretic therapy
B   Haemochromatosis
C   Primary hypoaldosteronism
D   Pancreatic carcinoma
E   Long-term steroid use

102. Non-accidental injury

Which one of the following is more likely to be an accidental than non-accidental injury?
A   Spiral fracture in the long bone of an infant
B   Sub-dural haematoma in a baby
C   Bruising on shins of a schoolboy
D   Tear of frenulum (central fold behind upper lip)
E   Multiple bruises of different ages

103. Haematology

The MCV (mean cell volume) is usually normal in which one of the following?
A   Iron deficiency anaemia
B   Chronic renal failure
C   Folate deficiency
D   Pernicious anaemia

104. Anaphylaxis

Which one of the following is not true? Anaphylaxis:
A   is mediated by IgE antibodies, which cause release of histamine and other vasoactive mediators
B   can be caused by antibiotics, NSAIDs, vaccines and blood
C   should be treated in the first instance with i.v. fluids such as sodium chloride
D   can be fatal

105. Generalised anxiety disorder

In the non-urgent treatment of generalised anxiety disorder in primary care, which one of the following is true?

A   To start treatment effectively, the diagnosis of GAD should not be rushed, as it can be stigmatising

B   If someone with diagnosed GAD does not improve after 'step 1' interventions, they should be offered high intensity psychological intervention or drug treatment

C   If a person with GAD chooses high intensity psychological intervention then applied relaxation can be offered

D   If a person with GAD chooses drug treatment then antipsychotics can be used in primary care

E   SNRI group of drugs should be considered first line

106. Practice accounts

Which one of the following is incorrect?

A   The GMS contract is the UK-wide contract between general practices and either NHS England or, in the rest of the UK, with the practice's primary care organisation

B   The GMS contract is made up of four main service elements including the global sum, the Quality and Outcomes framework and direct enhanced services

C   The global sum is made up of essential services and additional services

D   Enhanced services are not paid for within the global sum and can be directed or national

E   The global sum allocation is calculated using the Carr–Hill formula

F   When subletting rooms in the surgery premises, practices need to ensure that this income does not exceed 10% of the total gross NHS income to avoid an abatement of the practice's notional rent

107. Diabetic retinopathy

In the management of diabetic retinopathy, which one of the following does not require urgent referral (i.e. patient to be seen in seven days or less) to an ophthalmology specialist?

A   Rubeosis iridis is present

B   There is evidence of new vessel formation

C   There is sudden loss of vision

D   There are hard exudates within 1 disc diameter of the fovea

E   There is evidence of retinal detachment

108. Vitamin D

You are reviewing the blood results of a 73 year old lady who lives with her daughter and who has been complaining of weakness; her level of 25-hydroxyvitamin D (25-OHD) comes back as 60 nmol/l.

Which one of the following is true?

A   This level is optimal and no further action is required

B   This level is adequate; she requires lifestyle advice and should ensure she gets 400 IU per day through diet, sunshine and supplements

C   This level is indicative of vitamin D insufficiency; she requires high strength replacement for six weeks and then maintenance therapy

D   This lady has vitamin D deficiency so requires high strength replacement for ten weeks and then maintenance therapy

109–113. Headache

A Sub-arachnoid haemorrhage
B Cluster headache
C Trigeminal neuralgia
D Common migraine
E Ramsay Hunt Syndrome
F Giant cell arteritis
G Sub-dural haematoma

Match one of the conditions above to each of the scenarios below.

109. 56 year old woman complains of sudden severe electric-shock like episodes of pain affecting the left lower jaw – pain lasts 1–2 minutes each time then fades to a dull throb for a few hours; pain is provoked by laughing or chewing; mother had something similar.

110. 30 year old man who smokes 20 cigarettes a day presents with severe right-sided headache centred around right eye which is red and watery; pain lasts for an hour at time and is waking him from his sleep – has been going on for two days now; had a similar episode lasting a week approximately six months ago affecting the same side and has remained symptom-free until now. He thinks it may be related to drinking red wine.

111. A 28 year old mother attends complaining of recurrent episodes of one-sided throbbing headache; these occur every four weeks or so and are accompanied by nausea, vomiting and photophobia; she has had them since her teens but they are becoming worse now.

112. An 80 year old woman attends complaining of headache and scalp tenderness and blurred vision in her right eye; she denies jaw claudication or systemic upset; on examination her temporal arteries are pulsatile and tender; her ESR is raised.

113. A 38 year old man attends complaining of severe occipital headache – he describes feeling as though someone has hit him on the back of the head with a baseball bat; a few days ago he had a slight headache which he thought odd as he has never had a headache before.

114. Alcohol intake

Current guidelines suggest that men should drink no more than how much alcohol per week? (choose one answer only)

A 14 units
B 21 units
C 28 units
D 14 pints
E 21 pints
F 28 pints

115. Coeliac disease

With regard to coeliac disease, which one of the following statements is true?
A   The prevalence of coeliac disease in international population studies is 20%
B   Tissue transglutaminase antibody, endomysial antibody and immunoglobulin A should be used for initial testing
C   Unless antibodies are positive, coeliac disease cannot be diagnosed
D   Treatment involves a low carbohydrate diet, e.g. Atkins
E   Patients should be advised to start a gluten-free diet before any investigations are done
F   Patients should not be referred for further investigations unless antibody levels come back confirming coeliac disease

116. Gluten-free diet

Which one of the following products is gluten-free?
A   Rye
B   Semolina
C   Barley
D   Rice

117-122. Glycaemic index

Rate the GI index of the following foods as:
A   high
B   medium
C   low

117. White rice.

118. Sweetcorn.

119. Lucozade.

120. Cherries.

121. Pear.

122. Banana.

123. Diabetes diagnosis

Which one of the following is diagnostic of diabetes mellitus, based on the WHO diagnostic criteria?

A A 54 year old female who is asymptomatic and has a fasting blood glucose of 7.2 mmol/l and 7.1 mmol/l when repeated a week later

B A 54 year old female who is asymptomatic but has a single fasting blood glucose of 7.9 mmol/l

C A 54 year old female with a three month history of polyuria, polydipsia and a single fasting plasma glucose of 6.9 mmol/l

D A 54 year old female with a two month history of polyuria, polydipsia and repeated fasting blood glucose on three separate occasions of 6.9 mmol/l

E A 54 year old female with a three month history of polyuria, polydipsia and a single random blood sugar of 11.0 mmol/l

124-127. Vaginal discharge

A Herpes
B Candida
C Trichomoniasis
D Bacterial vaginosis
E Physiological
F Foreign body

Match the scenarios below to the diagnoses above – choose one in each case.

124. An Asian lady comes to see you, very distressed as she has developed a nasty vaginal discharge; she describes it as being very watery and grey. It is interfering with her ritual ablutions.

125. A young female student attends surgery complaining of a copious, mucopurulent, offensive, frothy green discharge; she thinks she may have a water infection as it is very sore to pass urine.

126. A heavily pregnant lady attends surgery worried about a heavy vaginal discharge; she describes it as having no odour, and as being thick and creamy, like cottage cheese.

127. A 26 year old married lady attends surgery with high fever and myalgia; she has multiple painful sores on the perineal mucosa and is finding it very difficult to pass urine because of the pain.

128-131. Aromatherapy

A   Indigestion
B   Insomnia, anxiety
C   Burns, relaxation
D   Clearing blocked noses

Match the aromatherapy oil below with its common use (choose only one in each case):

128. Lavender.

129. Valerian.

130. Peppermint.

131. Eucalyptus.

132. Hypokalaemia

Causes of hypokalaemia include all except which one of the following?
A   Long-term steroid use
B   Cushing's syndrome
C   Conn's syndrome
D   Addison's disease
E   Intestinal fistula

133. Hyponatraemia

Causes of hyponatraemia include all of the following except which one?
A   Diabetes insipidus
B   Addison's disease
C   Polydipsia
D   Diarrhoea / vomiting
E   Renal failure

134-139. Gynaecomastia

A Cancer bronchus
B Thyrotoxicosis
C Physiological
D Drug-related
E Liver disease
F Klinefelter's syndrome
G Testicular tumours

For each case presented below, choose one from the list of common causes of gynaecomastia above.

134. A 26 year old man is attending, worried about breast swelling and tenderness; on examination the breast area is enlarged and slightly tender; he is also tender over his epigastrium and when questioned admits to taking his father's cimetidine, which he has found helpful in relieving an ongoing problem with indigestion.

135. A 37 year old teacher attends surgery; he is very anxious as he has developed enlarged swollen breast tissue; he feels agitated all the time but assumes he is worried about an imminent school inspection and is not sleeping; he has also lost 7 kg in weight over the past 2 months; on examination you note he is clammy, his pulse is 106/minute and his blood pressure 140/80; he is currently taking bendrofluazide 2.5 mg once daily for hypertension.

136. A 20 year old student attends surgery having developed swelling affecting the breast area; he is otherwise fit and well; he drinks 28 units of alcohol per week and smokes 10–15 cigarettes per day; on examination you notice his left testis feels hard.

137. A 68 year old retired builder comes to see you as he is feeling generally unwell; he has lost 7 kg in weight over the past month and is generally off his food; on closer questioning he has had some chest discomfort but this is mainly localised to the breast area; he has had a tickly cough for a few weeks which is not settling; he has smoked 40/day since the age of 16 but recently has gone off them; he is on tablets for an ongoing problem with an enlarged prostate but cannot remember what they are called. On examination you note him to have clubbing of the fingers and there are decreased breath sounds on the left side; the percussion note is dull.

138. A young couple come to see you; they have been married for 2 years but have not managed to start a family yet; you note the husband is very tall; on examination he has painless breast enlargement and small testes.

139. A jolly 56 year old publican comes to see you; he has been getting some jokes from his customers for developing 'man boobs' and is wondering if he can be referred for surgery; he drinks and smokes with his customers but has no idea how much; on examination you notice multiple spider naevi over his chest and palpation of the abdomen reveals a sharply demarcated mass arising from under the right costal margin; notes reveal concerns regarding his LFTs.

140–146. DVLA and fitness to drive

A Refusal/revocation of licence
B 1 week off driving
C 4 weeks off driving
D 6 weeks off driving
E 11 months
F 12 months
G Permanently barred
H No driving restrictions

For each case presented, choose the correct length of time or other consequence in terms of driving licence from the choices above.

140. A 22 year old student attends surgery having recently been seen by the local neurologists for investigation of recurrent episodes of unconciousness; he has been told he has epilepsy and cannot drive; since being started on medication 1 month ago, he has been fit-free; he would like to know for how much longer he cannot drive.

141. A 68 year old retired school-mistress attends surgery; she had a single short-lived episode of weakness affecting the right hand 2 weeks ago; at the time she was also noted to have difficulty speaking and was slurring her words; her husband states that the whole episode lasted less than 10 minutes and she has been perfectly well since; she takes enalapril for hypertension and smokes 5 cigarettes per day.

142. A 44 year old housewife is worried about driving her child to school after she has had a pacemaker inserted next week; how long will she be unable to drive?

143. A 44 year old lorry driver is wondering whether it is ok for him to continue driving after his pacemaker insertion next week; you advise him, 'No.' How long will he be unable to drive for?

144. A 38 year old bus driver is diagnosed as being HIV positive.

145. A 59 year old lady has had a myocardial infarction; her husband attends surgery and informs you she is to have a CABG later that day; he would like to know how long she is likely to need off driving.

146. A 40 year old man is colour blind and has a visual acuity of 6/9 in both eyes.

147. Antibiotic prophylaxis

Which one of the following scenarios requires antibiotic prophylaxis?

A A 50 year old lady with a past history of infective endocarditis having a cervical smear

B A 60 year old man with a prosthetic heart valve *in situ* having a blood test

C A 36 year old lady with past history of infective endocarditis having a routine IUCD insertion 6 weeks after a normal vaginal delivery

D A heavily pregnant, anaemic lady found to have a previously undiagnosed murmur, due to have a dental extraction

E A 22 year old female student who wishes to have a pinna and nipple piercing on the same date

148. Notifiable diseases

All of the following are notifiable under the Public Health (Control of Disease) Act 1984 except which one?

A Mumps

B Measles

C HIV

D Dysentery

E Tuberculosis

149. Head lice

The following are true of head lice except which one?

A They typically affect the scalp with a predilection for the nape of the neck and behind the ears

B Key findings of a large European study concluded that being from a family of lower social class, having more siblings and longer hair, increased chances of having head lice

C Salicylate emulsion is helpful in their management

D Using a louse comb is more effective for detection of infestation than visual inspection alone

E Dimeticone treatment is considered effective

150. Glaucoma

The following are all important signs of glaucoma, except which one?

A Visual field constriction

B Increased intraocular pressure

C Proptosis

D Severe pain affecting eye

Answers to questions 101–150

101. Answer is C.

Hypoaldosteronism leads to raised blood pressure and low potassium; most are caused by an aldosterone-secreting adenoma.

102. Answer is C.

Spiral fractures are often the result of a twisting force being applied to a limb; the frenulum can be torn if a child has a dummy (pacifier) or bottle pushed aggressively into the mouth; bruises or injuries of different ages indicate that the abuse has been going on for some time, rather than being an isolated incident. (*NICE CG89, When to suspect child maltreatment*, December 2009).

103. Answer is B.

The MCV is decreased in iron deficiency anaemia and increased in pernicious anaemia and folate deficiency.

104. Answer is C.

Recent guidelines from the Resuscitation Council have emphasised early treatment with intramuscular adrenaline is the treatment of choice for an anaphylactic reaction. Obviously, the exact treatment will depend on the patient's location, the equipment and drugs available, and the skills of those treating the anaphylactic reaction, but oxygen and i.v. fluids should be given as soon as possible and antihistamines and steroids after the initial resuscitation (*Emergency treatment of anaphylactic reactions: guidelines for healthcare providers*, Working Group of the Resuscitation Council (UK), January 2008. This guidance should be read in conjunction with *NICE CG134*, Dec 2011, *Initial assessment and referral following emergency treatment for an anaphylactic episode*).

105. Answer is C.

The diagnosis of GAD should be identified and communicated as early as possible to help people understand the disorder and start effective treatment promptly; if someone with diagnosed GAD does not improve after 'step 1' interventions they should be offered low intensity psychological interventions such as individual guided or non-facilitated self-help in the first instance.

If a person with GAD chooses high intensity psychological intervention then either cognitive behavioural therapy or applied relaxation can be offered.

If a person with GAD chooses drug treatment then an SSRI should be offered; antipsychotics or benzodiazepines should not be used in primary care.

See *NICE Guidance CG113, Generalised anxiety disorder and panic disorder (with or without agoraphobia) in adults* (January 2011). This clinical guidance updates and replaces NICE Guidelines *CG22, Anxiety* (published December 2004; amended April 2007).

106. Answer is B.

There are three main service elements as noted (Tudor, A. (2013) *Practice Accounts Made Easy* – Chapter 8).

107. Answer is D.

Diabetic retinopathy is the leading cause of blindness in people under 60 in industrialised nations. It is also a major cause of blindness in older people. Twenty years after the onset of type 2 diabetes, over 60% of sufferers will have diabetic retinopathy but many will be asymptomatic until the disease is very advanced. The risk of visual impairment and blindness is reduced by care that combines screening with effective treatment. Screening must identify those with sight-threatening retinopathy that requires immediate preventative treatment.

If there is a sudden loss of vision the NICE guidelines on the management of diabetic retinopathy (published in 2002) recommend that the patient be seen within 24 hours by an ophthalmology specialist. This is also the case if there is evidence of retinal detachment. If new vessel formation, rubeosis iridis, or pre-retinal and/or vitreous haemorrhage is detected, patients should be seen within one week. An unexplained drop in visual acuity, hard exudates within one disc diameter of the fovea, macular oedema, unexplained retinal findings and pre-proliferative (or more advanced) retinopathy should be seen by a specialist within a maximum of four weeks.

108. Answer is B.

Vitamin D is a 'hot topic.' The table below helps guide management based on serum 25-OHD concentrations (*BMJ*, 2010; **340:** b5664).

Serum 25-OHD concentration	Vitamin D status	Manifestation	Management
<25 nmol/l	Deficient	Rickets Osteomalacia	Treat with high-dose calciferol
25–50 nmol/l	Insufficient	Associated with disease risk	Vitamin D supplementation
50–75 nmol/l	Adequate	Healthy	Lifestyle advice
>75 nmol/l	Optimal	Healthy	None

Questions 109–113: Answers given below, but SIGN published guidelines on the diagnosis and management of headache in adults (No. 107) in November 2008 which are useful reading, especially for questions 110, 111 and 113.

109. Answer is C.

TN (also known as tic douloureux) – paroxysmal bursts of severe burning or shock-like pain lasting from a few seconds to up to two minutes at a time;

typically felt on one side of the jaw or cheek; asymptomatic in-between attacks which can last from a few days up to months; triggers for attacks include chewing, laughing, shaving or being exposed to the wind; most often in people >50, f>m; can run in families perhaps because of an inherited pattern of blood vessel formation – ? an abnormal blood vessel pressing on trigeminal nerve. Treatment options include medication (anticonvulsants, tricyclics), complementary (acupuncture, biofeedback), and surgery; *NICE* (IPG085, August 2004) approved stereotactic surgery for TN using the gamma knife.

110. Answer is B.

A BMJ clinical review of cluster headache confirmed conventional analgesia is ineffective and not worth trying; it suggested instead to offer all patients short burst oxygen therapy and parenteral (injectable or nasal) triptans to treat attacks.

Preventative treatment options include a tapering dose of steroids or verapamil as the drug of choice (*BMJ*, 2012; **344**: e2407).

111. Answer is D.

The New Generalist (Volume 3, Autumn 2005) states that a stratified care approach where the patient receives the treatment most appropriate to their illness severity and frequency is preferable to the traditional step care analgesic approach: all patients will require acute medications (analgesics +/– anti-emetic for mild/moderate, triptan for moderate/severe) in the first instance; prophylaxis may be required for those with frequent (>3–4 attacks/month), disabling attacks, or for those who find acute medications ineffective/intolerable; first-line prophylactic agent likely to be a beta blocker in most cases (neuromodulators such as topiramate, amitriptyline, and calcium channel blockers also used but not all are licensed for this use in the UK).

Some complementary medications such as feverfew, magnesium, vitamin B2 (riboflavin), acupuncture and butterbur may be used in *addition to, but not instead of* usual medication (*MIPCA Guidelines*).

112. Answer is F.

Giant cell arteritis with neuro-ophthalmic complications requires a temporal artery biopsy as soon as possible to provide a tissue diagnosis to justify the long-term systemic steroid therapy (and its associated side-effects) that this condition requires, and also to help exclude other diagnoses, e.g. stroke. Treatment with high dose steroids initially and gradually reducing can take between six months and a year, or longer (*Br J Ophthalmol*, 2001; **85**: 1248–51).

113. Answer is A.

Sub-arachnoid haemorrhage is usually due to a bleed from an aneurysm and accounts for 5% of all strokes; half of patients are <55 years old and outcome is generally poor: it has a high mortality (50% die within a month) and morbidity (of survivors, 50% become dependent in terms of help with ADL – activities of daily living).

114. Answer is B.

Current recommendations are no more than 14 units for women and 21 for men.

115. Answer B is true.

Coeliac disease prevalence is 0.5–1% in international studies. Antibody-negative coeliac disease with villous atrophy is now recognised as a disease entity and patients who remain symptomatic despite negative blood tests should be referred for further testing; patients in whom coeliac disease is suspected should avoid starting a gluten-free diet until diagnostic confirmation with duodenal biopsy (*NICE Guidance CG86; Coeliac disease: recognition and assessment of coeliac disease*, May 2009).

116. Answer is D.

Rice, tapioca and sago are gluten-free, but wheat, barley, semolina and rye all contain gluten.

117. Answer is A.

118. Answer is B.

119. Answer is A.

120. Answer is C.

121. Answer is C.

122. Answer is B.

The glycaemic index is a numerical system that tells you how fast a particular food triggers a rise in your blood sugar levels; the higher the GI, the faster that particular food will cause a rise in blood sugar; for people such as diabetics, eating lower GI foods is thought to be beneficial by allowing a steady release of sugar into the bloodstream, reducing the need for snacking and helping with weight loss.

123. Answer is A.

Methods and criteria for diagnosing diabetes mellitus are as follows:

1. Diabetes symptoms (i.e. polyuria, polydipsia and unexplained weight loss) plus
a random venous plasma glucose concentration >11.1 mmol/l

or

a fasting plasma glucose concentration >7.0 mmol/l (whole blood >6.1 mmol/l) or

two hour plasma glucose concentration >11.1 mmol/l two hours after 75 g anhydrous glucose in an oral glucose tolerance test (OGTT).

2. If patient is asymptomatic, diagnosis should not be based on a single glucose determination but requires confirmatory plasma venous determination. At least one additional glucose test result on another day with a value in the diabetic range is essential, either fasting, from a random sample or from the two hour post glucose load. If the fasting or random values are not diagnostic the two hour value should be used.

Impaired fasting glycaemia is diagnosed on a fasting blood glucose level of 6.1–6.9 mmol/l.

This is an area which has come up a number of times in past AKT papers and one where the RCGP has advised that candidates should carefully review as it is likely to come up in future papers.

See www.sign.ac.uk/pdf/sign116.pdf, *Management of diabetes* (March 2010); World Health Organization (WHO) and International Diabetes Federation (IDF) (2006). *Definition and diagnosis of diabetes mellitus and intermediate hyperglycaemia* (www.who.int/diabetes/publications/Definition%20and%20 diagnosis%20of%20diabetes); www.diabetes.org.uk.

Questions 124–127. Answers drawn from *BMJ*, 2004; **328**: 1306–8.

124. Answer is D.
Ritual ablutions (or wudu) include washing of the perineal area with water; any discharge breaks the wudu, and soils the clothing, and so the patient has to perform the whole process again in order to enter a state of prayer. Treatment options include: metronidazole (oral, topical) or clindamycin (note: intravaginal clindamycin can cause condom failure, and because it also kills lacto bacilli can predispose to vulvovaginal candidiasis). Note also that relapse is common; the bacteria responsible do not persist in male partner and so treatment of male partner does not affect relapse rate.

125. Answer is C.

Symptoms of infection with the flagellated protozoan *Trichomonas vaginalis*, can also include vulvar irritation and superficial dyspareunia; transmission is usually sexual; external genital examination may be normal (classic strawberry cervix appearance due to punctate haemorrhage is uncommon); treatment options include oral metronidazole or tinidazole; side-effects of metronidazole include nausea, metallic taste in mouth, disulfiram reaction with alcohol so problems with compliance with lower dose and longer course regimens, although WHO prefers 5 day course for men, rather than single stat dose of 2 g; patient needs follow-up for test of cure and contact tracing.

126. Answer is B.

Candida infection is common; affects 75% women during their reproductive life; is associated with diabetes, pregnancy (or both!), antibiotic use and immunosuppression; transmission is mostly non-sexual; patient may present with external dysuria, superficial dysparuenia, as well as classic cottage cheese discharge; a large number of oral and topical preparations are available. Note that miconazole and econazole have an adverse effect on latex condoms so can cause condom failure.

127. Answer is A.

Herpes is the leading cause of genital ulcer disease worldwide (*BMJ*, 2007; **334**: 1048–52); counselling of patient and partner is very important; presentation of first episode is often severe and associated with systemic upset; urinary symptoms can be severe enough to include urinary retention; attacks can be managed symptomatically and antivirals such as acyclovir are recommended: they do not cure the illness but can reduce viral shedding and severity of illness; patient should be advised to use barrier method and avoid sexual intercourse when symptomatic; oral sex should be avoided when a cold sore is present.

The patient or her partner may have been carrying the virus and been asymptomatic for now, so this current event need not necessarily be a sign of infidelity.

For further information see: www.herpes.org.uk.

128. Answer is C.

Lavender can be used to aid relaxation and to help relieve pain and assist healing of burns.

129. Answer is B.

Valerian is useful in insomnia (also available in tablet form for oral use).

130. Answer is A.

Peppermint is useful for indigestion; and is used in the oral form to help with indigestion and bloating.

131. Answer is D.

Eucalyptus oil is very useful for clearing congestion.

132. Answer is D.

Addison's disease causes hyperkalaemia.

Other causes of hypokalaemia include diarrhoea, vomiting, purgative abuse.

Causes of hyperkalaemia include renal failure, ACE inhibitors, potassium-sparing diuretics.

133. Answer is A.

Diabetes insipidus causes an increase in sodium levels.

134. Answer is D.

Cimetidine, spironolactone and verapamil are all associated with an increased risk of gynaecomastia; the anti-ulcer drugs ranitidine and misoprostol are not (*BNF*, September 2009).

135. Answer is B.

Although thyrotoxicosis is more common in women than men, it can occur in men where it can cause the classic symptoms as described, as well as gynaecomastia and sexual dysfunction.

136. Answer is G.

The incidence of gynaecomastia in adult men is reported as being 35–65% depending on criteria used; 2% of men presenting with gynaecomastia are found to have testicular tumours; it is important to do a testicular examination on all men presenting with breast enlargement and advise those with a normal examination to continue to self-check regularly and report any abnormalities to their GP (*BMJ*, 2006; **332**: 837–8).

137. Answer is A.

This man has lung cancer and a pleural effusion on the left side; the tumour is releasing chemicals that are causing gynaecomastia – this is known as a paraneoplastic syndrome.

138. Answer is F.

Men with Klinefelter's syndrome may have breast enlargement; they also tend to have testicular atrophy and be azoospermic.

139. Answer is E.

This man has signs of liver failure secondary to chronic excess alcohol consumption.

140. Answer is E.

Note that he was started on medication 1 month ago and has been fit-free since; hence only 11 months to go!

141. Answer is C.

The DVLA (March 2013) states that a patient having a single TIA must not drive for at least one month and may resume after this time if the clinical recovery is satisfactory (www.dft.gov.uk/dvla).

142. Answer is B.

Pacemaker implant (includes box change): driving must cease for at least one week; may be permitted thereafter provided there is no other disqualifying condition.

143. Answer is D.

Pacemaker implant disqualifies Group 2 driver for 6 weeks. Re-licensing may be permitted thereafter provided there is no other disqualifying condition.

144. Answer is H.

HIV is not a bar to driving either a group 1 or group 2 vehicle.

145. Answer is C.

CABG: driving must cease for 4 weeks – may resume thereafter provided no other disqualifying condition exists; DVLA do not need to be notified.

146. Answer is H.

Colour blindness is not a bar to driving a group 1 or group 2 vehicle; visual acuity must be satisfactory in both colour blind and normal-sighted persons equally.

147. Answer is C.

For gynaecological procedures, it is recommended that antibiotic prophylaxis is given to women with prosthetic valves or who have had endocarditis previously; in these circumstances an intravenous regimen is advised; in the absence of specific guidance the FFPRHC considers that such prophylaxis should be used for both insertion and removal (*NICE Long Acting Reversible Contraception: CG30*, Oct 2005).

NICE Guidance CG64 (March 2008, *Prophylaxis against infective endocarditis: antimicrobial prophylaxis against infective endocarditis in adults and children undergoing interventional procedures*) states that women undergoing procedures to the genitourinary tract (including urological, gynaecological and obstetric procedures, and childbirth) should not be offered antibiotic prophylaxis against infective endocarditis.

Therefore, cervical smear does not require antibiotic prophylaxis, nor does routine phlebotomy or dental procedures.

The murmur in the pregnant lady is probably a flow murmur.

The guidelines for the prevention of endocarditis: report of the Working Party of the British Society for Antimicrobial Chemotherapy (Gould *et al.* (2006) *J Antimicrob Chem*) states that where the process involves non-infected skin incision but no mucosal breach (e.g. in the case of nipple or pinna piercings), antibiotic prophylaxis is not needed but adequate skin disinfection should be carried out prior to the procedure.

148. Answer is C.

It is a statutory obligation that a medical practitioner must report a notifiable disease to the Consultant responsible for Communicable Disease Control (see Public Health (Control of Disease) Act, 1984). These notifiable diseases include: acute encephalitis, acute poliomyelitis, anthrax, cholera, diphtheria, dysentery, food poisoning, leptospirosis, leprosy, malaria, measles, meningitis, mumps, ophthalmia neonatorum, paratyphoid fever, plague, rabies, relapsing fever, rubella, scarlet fever, smallpox, tetanus, typhus fever, viral haemorrhagic fever, viral hepatitis, whooping cough, yellow fever.

149. Answer C is false.

Do remember that, when treating an entire family, it is a legal requirement to issue one prescription per person (*Drugs and Therapeutic Bulletin*, July 2007).

150. Answer is C.

Proptosis is a forward displacement of the orbit and is not a sign of glaucoma.

Questions 151-200

for answers see pages 67–72

151-156. Herbal remedies

A Indigestion
B Migraine
C Depression
D Eczema
E Prevention and treatment of common cold and other viruses
F Insomnia

Match the herbal remedy below with its common use.

151. St John's Wort

152. Feverfew

153. Chinese herbal medicine

154. Echinacea

155. Peppermint

156. Valerian

157. Seborrhoeic warts

Which one of the following statements is true?
A Arise from the sebaceous glands
B Are common in people over the age of 50 years
C Are found mostly on the hands and face
D Are pre-malignant
E Are caused by a wart virus

158-166. Haematology

A Felty's syndrome
B Burkitt's lymphoma
C Non-Hodgkin's lymphoma
D Iron deficiency anaemia
E Chronic myeloid leukaemia
F Acute lymphoblastic leukaemia
G Chronic lymphocytic leukaemia
H Multiple myeloma
I Vitamin B12 deficiency
J Vitamin D deficiency
K Sickle cell disease
L Hodgkin's lymphoma

For each scenario described below, select the single most likely diagnosis from the list above.

158. A 35 year old man presents with weight loss, lassitude and anaemia; on examination you note he has a markedly enlarged spleen; investigations reveal anaemia, raised white cell count, positive Philadelphia chromosome.

159. A 28 year old nurse attends with her fiancé who is a medical registrar; they had noticed a solitary enlarged rubbery cervical lymph node in the right sub-mandibular region; they are concerned as she appears to be losing weight for no obvious reason and have come in today for the results of blood tests; the haematologist has remarked on the presence of Reed–Sternberg cells.

160. A 7 year old Sudanese boy presents with night sweats, fever, weight loss; his mother has noticed a mass arising from the left lower jaw; blood tests show a positive monospot.

161. A 70 year old man is awaiting surgery for his prostate; routine blood testing shows him to have a raised lymphocyte count. The haematologist has commented on the presence of 'smear cells' and has already made an outpatient appointment to see him.

162. A 60 year old man presents with a 6 week history of progressive mid-thoracic back pain and tenderness; the main reason for attending today is that he has not been able to shake a recent chest infection and every time he coughs, the pain in his back is exacerbated; you organise some blood tests and when they return, they show anaemia, raised ESR and rouleaux formation; serum electrophoresis shows a paraprotein band and urine electrophoresis confirms the presence of Bence-Jones proteins.

163. A 49 year old lady attends complaining of fatigue, a sore mouth and difficulty swallowing; she is also worried that she is losing hair and is wondering if you can give her anything for heavy periods.

164. A 36 year old vegan lady attends complaining of a sore mouth; you note her to have a smooth, sore tongue; she has numbness affecting her limbs in a 'glove and stocking' distribution; on examination her joint position and vibration sense are disturbed.

165. A 4 year old boy presents with fever, weight loss, and severe bilateral leg pains; he bruises easily and is suffering from recurrent chest infections; full blood count shows a pancytopenia.

166. A 7 year old boy of Afro-Caribbean descent presents with severe abdominal pain and swelling of the hands and feet; blood film shows presence of elongated crescent-shaped blood cells.

167. Disability Living Allowance

With regard to changes in 2013 to Disability Living Allowance, which one of the following is untrue?

A This is being replaced by personal independence payments (PIP) for those aged 16 to 64

B Those who have been awarded a lifetime or indefinite award will be unaffected

C The PIP award comprises the daily living and mobility components, each of which is split into a standard and enhanced rate

D The allowance is based on how an illness affects a person rather than the diagnosis itself

168. Semen analysis

Which one of the following is false?

A Collection is by masturbation after abstinence from sexual activities, including masturbation for 3–5 days

B The sample is not tested for sperm antibodies

C If the first sample is abnormal, patients should be referred immediately with a view to sperm recovery and cryopreservation

D The sample must be taken to lab as soon as possible after production and be kept warm during transfer

169. Irritable bowel syndrome

Which one of the following is true regarding irritable bowel syndrome?

A Typically presents in the over 50s

B FBC, ESR or CRP are not helpful in diagnosis and should not be performed as they are not recommended to exclude other diagnostic possibilities

C In management, insoluble fibre (bran) is more helpful than soluble fibre (ispaghula powder)

D May respond to small doses of amitriptyline

E Acupuncture and reflexology should be encouraged by primary care physicians as a means of self help

F Is a diagnosis of exclusion using Dukes' classification

170. Atopic eczema

Considering emollient therapy, which one of the following is true?

A Bath emollients can cause allergic contact dermatitis

B There is strong evidence to support the use of bath emollients over topical emollients

C There is no general consensus amongst clinicians to confirm that the application of emollients directly to the skin is effective

D The routine use of antiseptic/emollient preparations in patients with atopic eczema is highly recommended

171. Diabetes mellitus

Which one of the following statements is true?

A Poor glycaemic control at conception and during pregnancy is associated with an increased risk of stillbirth

B Symptoms alone (e.g. subjective feelings of weakness) are a very good indicator of biochemical hypoglycaemia (blood glucose <3 mmol/l)

C In the case of a diabetic patient with COPD, extra blood glucose monitoring is not necessary during intercurrent infections, as long as any such exacerbations are treated with a course of oral prednisolone

D NICE guidelines for patients with type II diabetes, suggest that self-monitoring of blood glucose levels can be considered a stand-alone intervention

172. Therapeutics

You are reviewing the blood results for the day and note that one of your diabetic patients' creatinine is 140 µmol/l. You arrange to see him to review the dose.

At what level of creatinine should metformin be stopped?

A 130 µmol/l

B 140 µmol/l

C 150 µmol/l

D 160 µmol/l

173. Impetigo

A 4 year old boy is brought in with a lesion on the right cheek, about the size of a two pence piece, which has been present for 2 days; it started off as an insect bite when he had been at his grandmother's; this then blistered, broke down, and the liquid dried to a golden brown crust; he is otherwise well and has had all his immunisations to date.

Which one of the following statements should you make to the mother?
A   Current evidence shows that removing the crust and applying topical antiseptics is the treatment of choice and is highly effective
B   Not to worry, as the condition is not very contagious
C   His teachers are likely to be perfectly happy for him to continue to attend school
D   You need to contact social workers as this is a case of non-accidental injury
E   The condition usually leaves permanent hyper-pigmentation and scarring
F   He may need antibiotics

174-178. Evidence-based medicine: studies

Consider the following types of study and put them in hierarchical order of evidence starting with (for question 174) the study that carries the greatest weight, and ending (for question 178) with the study that carries the least weight.
A   Expert committee reports
B   High quality case-control study
C   Reasonably high quality randomised controlled trials
D   Cohort study with high risk of bias
E   High quality meta-analysis of randomised controlled trials

179-189. Statistical terms and studies

A Mode
B Mean
C Median
D Case-control
E Cross-sectional
F Cohort
G Confidence interval
H Attributable risk
I Relative risk
J Number needed to treat
K None of these
M Meta analysis

Match the definition to one of the options given above.

179. The sum of all the values given, divided by the number of values.

180. The mid-point of a given set of values such that half are below, half are above.

181. The most commonly occurring value.

182. A range, within which we can be fairly certain that the true value lies.

183. A descriptive study that provides a snapshot of the population being studied.

184. A prospective observational study that follows a group over a period of time and investigates the effect of a treatment or risk factor; can calculate incidence of a disease.

185. A retrospective study which investigates the relationship between a risk factor and one or more outcomes; carried out by selecting cases that already have disease, matching them to cases who are the same but disease-free, and then comparing the effect of the risk factor on the two groups. It looks for exposure and can be used to calculate the odds ratio.

186. Incidence of disease in exposed population divided by incidence of disease in non-exposed population.

187. Incidence of disease in exposed population minus incidence of disease in non-exposed population.

188. Reciprocal of attributable risk.

189. A method of combining results from a number of independent studies to give one overall estimate of benefit or harm in the forms of an odds ratio.

190-192. Cremation forms

A   Form A
B   Form B
C   Form C

Match the form correctly to each scenario below.

190. Certificate of medical attendant to be signed by first doctor.

191. Application for cremation.

192. Signed by a second doctor who is not in partnership with the first doctor and who has been qualified for at least 5 years.

193. Chlamydia

The following are all suitable options for treating chlamydia except which one?
A   Azithromycin 1 g stat.
B   Doxycycline 100 mg b.d. 1 week
C   Erythromycin 500 mg b.d. 2 weeks
D   Topical clindamycin

194-198. Hypertension

A   Angiotensin-converting enzyme inhibitor
B   Calcium-channel blocker
C   Thiazide diuretic
D   Beta-blocker
E   Angiotensin II receptor antagonists
F   Thiazide-like diuretic

Consider the following hypertensive patients, all of whom need treatment and, bearing recent evidence and guidelines in mind, suggest the single best class of anti-hypertensive for each patient from the list above.

194. A 40 year old Caucasian lady.

195. A 60 year old Caucasian man with a past history of gout.

196. A 40 year old man of Afro-Caribbean origin, also with a history of gout.

197. A 55 year old man who also suffers with angina.

198. A patient who was initially on enalapril but has a troublesome tickly cough.

199. TIA

A 72 year old gentleman with well-controlled hypertension attends your clinic, giving a 30 minute history of slurred speech and weakness in his right arm the previous evening from which he has now fully recovered.

Which one of the following scoring systems would most help you manage him?

A ABCD2

B Wells criteria

C FAST

D $CHADS_2$

E PHQ-9

200. Confidence intervals

If a study quotes a 95% confidence interval, which one of the following statements is true?

A There is a 95% chance of the true value lying outside these limits

B There is a 5% chance of the true value lying outside these limits

C There is a 2.5% chance of the true value lying outside these limits

D There is a minus 5% chance of the true value lying outside these limits

Answers to questions 151–200

151. Answer is C.
A meta analysis of 23 RCTs shows St John's Wort is more effective than placebo and as effective as conventional antidepressants in mild to moderate depression, with fewer side-effects; significant interactions have been reported, especially with SSRIs, warfarin and COCP. There is now evidence that hypericum in doses of 900 mg is at least as effective as 20 mg paroxetine in moderate to severe depression and is better tolerated; physicians, however, are not encouraged to promote it but should be aware that many people do self prescribe OTC (*BMJ* 2005; **330**: 503–6).

152. Answer is B.
Both *Bandolier* and *Cochrane Database* (Pittler *et al.* 2000: Feverfew for preventing migraine) have stated that studies show that feverfew may be beneficial for the prevention of migraine; its effectiveness has not been established beyond reasonable doubt; adverse effects are minimal. Furthermore, the *Migraine in Primary Care Guidelines* have stated that complementary therapies such as feverfew, magnesium, vitamin B2, acupuncture and butterbur may be used in addition to, but not instead of, regular medication (www.mipca.org.uk/guidelines_mig.htm, 2006).

153. Answer is D.
Chinese herbal medicine is based on principles of yin and yang and aims to treat ill health through re-balancing these two elements and so allow the person's Qi to flow, thus restoring health; it has been used to treat a number of conditions, including skin disease.

154. Answer is E.
Echinacea, in a double-blind study, has been shown to be ineffective against the common cold (*NEJM*, 2005; **353**: 341–8). *Bandolier* and the *Cochrane Database* reported similar thoughts in 2000; however, many people do take this preparation OTC with or without zinc and vitamin C.

155. Answer is A.
Peppermint is used in many indigestion remedies both prescribed and OTC.

156. Answer is F.
Valerian is used in many stress and sleep aids (e.g. Kalms).

157. Answer is B.
Seborrhoeic warts are benign greasy-brown warty lesions, usually on back, chest, face and are very common in the elderly.

158. Answer is E.

CML is most commonly seen in middle age, often with a male preponderance; symptoms are chronic and insidious; those without the Philadelphia chromosome have a poorer prognosis.

159. Answer is L.

Lymphomas are a malignant proliferation of lymphocytes; Hodgkin's lymphomas are characterised by cells with mirror-image nuclei – the Reed–Sternberg cells; tend to occur as painless enlarged nodes.

160. Answer is B.

Burkitt's lymphoma: endemic across certain regions of equatorial Africa; high-grade B cell neoplasm; endemic African form most often affects maxilla or mandible; sporadic (non-endemic) form tends to affect abdominal organs; Epstein–Barr virus has been implicated strongly in endemic form, relationship less clear with sporadic form; mean age in Africa: 7.

161. Answer is G.

25% of patients with CLL are asymptomatic; prognosis is good; affects elderly.

162. Answer is H.

Postural bone pain and tenderness is common in this neoplastic proliferation of plasma cells with diffuse bone marrow infiltration and focal osteolytic lesions; can present as pathological fracture; X-rays may show punched-out lesions (pepper pot skull). Multiple myeloma affects elderly.

163. Answer is D.

This lady has iron deficiency anaemia, which has led to angular cheilosis (fissures at angles of mouth), atrophic glossitis (smooth tongue) and the Plummer–Vinson (or Patterson–Kelly–Brown) syndrome of incoordinate movements in the pharynx, sometimes accompanied by actual web formation which causes dysphagia.

164. Answer is I.

This lady is deficient in vitamin B12 and has sub-acute combined degeneration of the spinal cord.

165. Answer is F.

Pancytopenia in a 4 year old boy is ALL.

166. Answer is K.

The crescent-shaped blood cells have 'sickled'; the child is suffering from hand and foot syndrome.

167. Answer is B.

168. Answer is C.

NICE Guidance CG156 (February 2013) *Fertility: assessment and treatment for people with fertility problems* states that if the first sample is abnormal, it should be repeated after 3 months to allow time for a cycle of spermatozoa formation to be completed.

Sperm antibodies are produced by the female; NICE states that screening for sperm antibodies should not be offered as there is no effective treatment to improve fertility.

169. Answer is D.

IBS typically presents in the 20–40 age group; Manning's criteria is helpful in diagnosis, which is one of exclusion (Dukes' classification is used for staging of colorectal adenocarcinoma). Initial investigations like FBC, ESR, CRP may be helpful in excluding sinister causes for symptoms. *NICE Guidance CG61, Irritable bowel syndrome in adults: diagnosis and management of irritable bowel syndrome in primary care* (February 2008).

170. Answer is A.

Although emollient bath additives are often prescribed for the treatment of eczema and related disorders, the evidence base for their use is not strong (*Drug and Therapeutics Bulletin*, October 2007).

171. Answer is A.

It is very important for women of child-bearing age who are diabetic to have antenatal counselling to avoid a poor perinatal outcome (*Drug and Therapeutics Bulletin*, September 2007).

NICE CG63 (March 2008, reissued July 2008, *Diabetes in pregnancy: management of diabetes and its complications from pre-conception to the postnatal period*) confirms this and states that women with diabetes who are planning to become pregnant should be offered pre-conception care (e.g. 5 mg folic acid, and renal assessment including microalbuminuria) and advice before discontinuing contraception.

172. Answer is C.

Metformin should be stopped if the creatinine is >150 µmol/l or the eGFR is <30 ml/min/1.73m^2.

173. Answer is F.

There is insufficient evidence to show whether removing crust or using topical antiseptics is likely to be helpful.

Topical fucidic acid for 7 days as a first-line treatment is a reasonable option; however, there is a growing problem with *Staph. aureus* resistance in the community in which case topical mupirocin may be considered, but only if the cause is MRSA.

Oral flucloxacillin may be needed if the infection is crusted and extensive, or bullous in nature. If streptococcal infection is known or suspected, phenoxymethylpenicillin can be added to flucloxacillin (*Drug and Therapeutics Bulletin*, January 2007).

174. Answer is E.
The study with the greatest weight in terms of evidence-based medicine is a high quality meta-analysis of randomised controlled trials.

175. Answer is C.
Next is a reasonably high quality RCT.

176. Answer is B.
Then a high quality case-control study.

177. Answer is D.
A cohort study with a high risk of bias is less good.

178. Answer is A.
An expert committee report is regarded as having the weakest evidence base.

179. Answer is B.
The mean of the numbers 5, 6, 6, 6, 7, 9, 10 is $(5+6+6+6+7+9+10)/7 = 49/7 = 7$.

180. Answer is C.
The median of the set of numbers above is 6.

181. Answer is A.
The mode (most frequently occurring number or event) of the same set of numbers is 6.

182. Answer is G.
If the confidence interval is 95%, we can be 95% certain that the true value lies within these limits.

183. Answer is E.
A cross-section at a point in time, e.g. undertaking a survey to see prevalence of chlamydia in a population.

184. Answer is F.
For example, a cohort study in the *BJGP* in 2004 looked at the fat intake in a group of newly diagnosed non-insulin dependent diabetics over a (prospective, moving forwards) 4 year period and found that, at diagnosis, many had an unfavourable fat intake, but that soon after, a majority adopted a more favourable consumption pattern and this improved pattern was maintained over the 4 year period.

185. Answer is D.

For example, looking back (retrospective), the use of thalidomide is compared between a group of women having abnormal babies and those having healthy ones.

186. Answer is I.

For example, if the risk of developing a DVT on pill A is 24/1000 and the risk on pill B was 8/1000, then the relative risk would be 0.024/0.008 = 3.

187. Answer is H.

For example, the incidence of disease X in smokers is 20% but the incidence in non-smokers is 2%; the attributable risk is 20%-2%=18%.

188. Answer is K.

189. Answer is M.

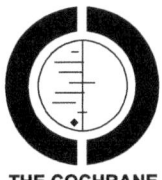

THE COCHRANE COLLABORATION®

For example, the Cochrane logo represents seven randomised controlled trials looking at the effect of antepartum glucocorticoid treatment to prevent respiratory distress syndrome in pre-term infants, something that was proven to be beneficial on meta analysis and is now routinely used.

The Cochrane logo is used here with permission.

190. Answer is B.

Form B can only be signed by a doctor who has attended the patient professionally within 14 days of death and has viewed the body after death; if the attending doctor is unavailable then a GP partner may sign form B.

191. Answer is A.

This form must be completed by the nearest surviving relative or executor; if this is not the case then a reason must be stated explaining this.

192. Answer is C.

Form C can only be signed by the second doctor once he has seen the body and discussed death with the first doctor, and preferably with someone who was present at the time of death (*Chief Medical Officer's Update 27*, May 2005).

Doctors filling in forms B and C should ensure that there is true independence between the two doctors completing forms A and B, that they have fully examined the body and discussed the case with each other; in addition, they should speak to a relative or other person who may have attended the deceased.

193. Answer is D.
Clindamycin is a treatment option for bacterial vaginosis, as is oral or topical metronidazole (unless pregnant in which case stick to clindamycin).

194. Answer is A.
ACE inhibitors are a good first-line choice in someone who is not black and who is less than age 55.

195. Answer is B.
Gout would be aggravated by thiazide and thiazide-like diuretics.

196. Answer is B.
Gout would be aggravated by thiazide and thiazide-like diuretics.

197. Answer is D.
WHO Guidelines state that beta blockers are still indicated in the treatment of hypertension for those patients who have had an MI or who suffer from angina; they are contraindicated in asthma, COPD, heart block, diabetes and heart failure.

198. Answer is E.
Angiotensin II receptor antagonists are useful for those patients who are bothered by cough while on ACE inhibitors (*British Hypertension Society, RCP, NICE CG127*; this clinical guideline (published in August 2011) updates and replaces NICE CG34 (June 2006).

199. Answer is A.
Wells criteria calculates pulmonary embolism and DVT probability score.

FAST is an acronym used as a mnemonic to help detect and enhance responsiveness to stroke victim needs.

$CHADS_2$ is a clinical prediction rule for estimating the risk of stroke in patients with non-rheumatic atrial fibrillation.

PHQ-9 refers to the nine-item depression scale of the Patient Health Questionnaire; it is a tool for assisting primary care clinicians in diagnosing depression as well as selecting and monitoring treatment.

200. Answer is B.
The 95% CI indicates that the true value has a 95% chance of lying within this range; it is represented on a Forrest Plot as a horizontal line; a longer line means a wider CI.

Questions 201-250

for answers see pages 83–87

201. Cataract

In the developing world cataracts are the number one cause of blindness, and surgery for them is the commonest operation; the following are all known risk factors except which one?

A   Malnutrition
B   Diabetes mellitus
C   Systemic steroids
D   UVB light
E   Gentamicin

202-207. Genetic inheritance

A   1 in 1
B   1 in 2
C   1 in 4
D   Definite
E   None of the above

Match the chance of developing the disease to each of the scenarios below.

202. Male child with both parents carriers for phenylketonuria.

203. Female child with both parents carriers for cystic fibrosis.

204. Male child of heterozygous mother carrying gene for haemophilia.

205. Female child of father with red–green colour blindness; mother is not a carrier.

206. Female child of father with red–green colour blindness; mother is a carrier.

207. Male child of parents where mother is known to have neurofibromatosis.

208. Illicit drug use during pregnancy

A 19 year old primip attends surgery for a routine antenatal test; she discloses that she regularly smokes cannabis with her boyfriend and would like to know if this is 'risky for the baby.'

Which one of the following is true?

A Smoking cannabis during pregnancy is associated with smaller birth weight
B Smoking cannabis during pregnancy is associated with gestational diabetes
C Smoking cannabis during pregnancy is associated with a decreased chance of miscarriage due to relaxed uterine tone
D Smoking cannabis during pregnancy is associated with macrosomia
E Smoking cannabis during pregnancy is associated with an increased risk of midline craniofacial defects

209-213. ENT

A Chronic secretory otitis media
B Acute otitis media with perforation
C Ramsay–Hunt syndrome
D Acoustic neuroma
E Otitis externa
F Tonsillitis

Match the diagnosis above to each of the following scenarios – each diagnosis may be used only once, or not at all.

209. A 26 year old man returns from holidaying in the Seychelles with his partner; he has a sore and itchy left ear.

210. A happy 6 year old boy, who has Down syndrome attends with bilateral conductive hearing loss.

211. A 45 year old lady presents with a right-sided lower motor neuron facial nerve palsy, imbalance and sensorineural deafness; on examination you note a crop of vesicles affecting the right ear canal.

212. A 20 year old man presents with progressive sensorineural deafness, vertigo and tinnitus affecting the right ear only.

213. A 16 year old girl presents with fever, malaise, headache and bilateral ear pain which is exacerbated by swallowing.

214. Treatment of varicose veins

Which one of the following is considered the optimal treatment for varicose veins in terms of cost-effectiveness?

A Conventional saphenofemoral ligation, stripping of long saphenous vein and phlebectomies

B Conventional sclerotherapy

C Foam sclerotherapy

D Phlebectomy

E Radio-frequency and laser ablation

215. Emergency referral for varicose veins

According to NICE, which one of the following scenarios warrants an emergency referral?

A A varicosity that has bled once and is in danger of bleeding again

B Bleeding from a varicosity that has eroded the skin

C An ulcer that is progressive and painful despite treatment

D Recurrent superficial thrombophlebitis

216. Thyrotoxicosis

The following are features of thyrotoxicosis except which one?

A Weight gain

B Palpitations

C Proximal myopathy

D Increased skin pigmentation

E Menstrual irregularities

217. Anaemia

Causes of a microcytic anaemia include all the following except which one?

A Iron deficiency

B Renal failure

C Anaemia of chronic disease

D Thalassaemia trait

E Pernicious anaemia

F Sideroblastic anaemia

218-220. Quality of life

A Barthel scale
B Modified Rankin score
C Mini-mental state examination

Match the scoring tool to its purpose. Each tool may be used once, more than once, or not at all.

218. A scale used to measure performance in activities of daily living (ADL). Each performance item is rated on this scale, with a given number of points assigned to each level or ranking. It uses ten variables describing ADL and mobility.

219. A commonly used scale for measuring the degree of disability or dependence in the daily activities of people who have suffered a stroke or other causes of neurological disability.

220. The scale runs from 0 (perfect health without symptoms) to 6 (death).

221. Vaginal bleeding

A 22 year old lady presents with moderate left iliac fossa pain and vaginal bleeding six weeks after her last period; her pulse is 72 b.p.m. and blood pressure is 120/80; she is apyrexial; she has a past history of pelvic inflammatory disease for which she last had antibiotics 6 months ago; she has no allergies; she was seen by one of your colleagues 4 days ago when a urine test confirmed pregnancy.

Choose the next single most appropriate step in this scenario.
A Advise bed rest and regular paracetamol until review by her own doctor tomorrow
B Congratulate her on her pregnancy and arrange routine booking for bloods and an ultrasound scan at 12 weeks
C Admit as a gynaecology emergency
D Treat recurrence of PID with clarithromycin and ciprofloxacin
E Arrange for high vaginal swabs and treat with clarithromycin and ciprofloxacin once causative agent confirmed

222. Psoriasis

Which one of the following statements regarding psoriasis is true?
A It is aggravated by sunlight
B It commonly spares intertriginous areas
C Plaques have diffuse edges
D It exhibits the phenomenon of koebnerisation
E NICE has recommended the use of tacrolimus for severe plaque psoriasis in adults who have failed to respond to standard systemic treatments

223–226. Drug interactions

A Cranberry juice
B Grapefruit juice
C Marmite
D Vodka

Match the foodstuff above with the drug it is likely to interact adversely with.

223. Disulfiram.

224. Moclobemide.

225. Simvastatin.

226. Warfarin.

227. Depression

For a 67 year old lady who had a myocardial infarction 8 months ago, and who presents with moderate depression, what would be your drug of choice?
A Venlafaxine
B Nortriptyline
C Sertraline
D Moclobemide
E Imipramine
F Omega-3 fatty acid supplementation

228. Rheumatoid arthritis

A 35 year old lady attends surgery giving a 10 week history of fatigue and bilateral pain and swelling affecting the small joints of her hands which are very stiff in the morning; blood tests show her to have a raised rheumatoid factor as well as inflammatory markers.

You feel she has rheumatoid arthritis. *Which one of the following is the first-line treatment for this condition?*

A Rest
B Simple pain killers such as paracetamol which she can buy herself
C Regular non-steroidal anti-inflammatory drugs with a proton pump inhibitor
D Urgent referral to secondary care for consideration of DMARD such as methotrexate

229. Alzheimer's dementia

The acetylcholinesterase inhibitors donepezil, galantamine and rivastigmine are recommended as options for mild to moderate Alzheimer's disease.

Memantine is recommended as an option in all but which one of the following?

A Mild Alzheimer's disease
B Severe Alzheimer's disease
C Moderate Alzheimer's disease where acetylcholinesterase inhibitors are contraindicated
D Moderate Alzheimer's disease where acetylcholinesterase inhibitors are not tolerated

230. Occupational lung disease

Which one of the following statements is correct?

A If a patient develops an occupational disease, their doctor is obliged to inform their employer in writing, with or without the patient's consent
B If a patient develops an occupational disease, their doctor is obliged to inform RIDDOR (Reporting of Injuries, Diseases and Dangerous Occurrences Regulations) with or without the patient's consent
C Pneumoconiosis (coal worker's lung) is not a notifiable disease
D Irritant dermatitis (hairdresser's hands) is a notifiable disease
E Industrial injuries disablement benefit is only payable if the effect of the injury lasts beyond the 91st day and the employee has to prove they were not to blame

231-235. HIV transmission

A   Zero risk
B   1 in 1000
C   1–3 in 100
D   1 in 300
E   5–10 in 100

Match the risk of infectivity with each exposure type described below.

231. Hugging an HIV-positive person.

232. Percutaneous exposure through needlestick injury.

233. Female having vaginal sexual intercourse with HIV-positive male.

234. Male having sexual intercourse with HIV-positive female.

235. HIV-infected urine splash in eye.

236-242. Consultation models

A Pendleton
B Roger Neighbour
C Byrne and Long
D Balint
E Eric Berne: transactional analysis
F Stott and Davis
G Helman
H Heron's interventional model
I Biomedical model

Match the description below to the single most appropriate consultation model.

236. Management of presenting complaint, management of ongoing problems, opportunistic health promotion, modification of health-seeking behaviour.

237. Connect, summarise, hand-over, safety-net, house-keeping.

238. What happened? Why? Why to me? Why now? What if I ignore it? What should I do?

239. Consultation can be instructive, informative, cathartic, confronting, supportive, catalytic.

240. History, examination, investigation, treatment.

241. This model introduced concept of heartsink patient, the doctor as a drug, the flash, the collusion of anonymity.

242. The games people play; roles of doctor and patient analysed in terms of role of parent, adult, child.

243-248. Chromosomal abnormalities

A 47XXY
B 45XO
C 5p deletion
D Trisomy 21
E Trisomy 18
F 46XX
G Trisomy 13

Match each of the phenotypes to one of the genotypes.

243. Flat occiput, low set eyes with prominent epicanthic folds, single palmar crease, congenital heart disease.

244. Males, tall stature, gynaecomastia, low IQ, infertility.

245. Rocker-bottom feet, low set ears, receding chin, developmental delay, index finger overlaps 3rd digit.

246. Females, broad chests with wide-spaced nipples, increased carrying angle at elbows, lymphoedema of hands and feet.

247. Normal phenotype.

248. Microcephaly, developmental delay, alert expression, abnormal cat-like cry, moon-shaped face, marked epicanthic folds.

249. Malaria

Considering non-drug preventative interventions in adult travellers, which one of the following is likely to be most beneficial?
A Acoustic buzzers
B Air conditioning and electric fans
C Smoke
D Insecticide-treated clothing and/or nets
E Aerosol insecticides

250. Statins

A 56 year old gentleman has been found to have raised cholesterol and you decide to start him on simvastatin.

Which one of the following is least likely to interact with it and cause a myositis?

A   Amlodipine
B   Cranberry juice
C   Bezafibrate
D   Clarithromycin

Answers to questions 201-250

201. Answer is E.

Gentamicin is ototoxic.

The main extrinsic factors associated with cataract formation in the developed world are smoking, diabetes and use of systemic steroids. Additional factors in the developing world include malnutrition, acute dehydrating disease and cumulative exposure to UVB sunlight (*BMJ*, 2006; **333**: 128–32).

202. Answer is C.

Phenylketonuria is inherited in an autosomal recessive manner.

203. Answer is C.

Cystic fibrosis is inherited in an autosomal recessive manner (as are sickle cell disease and glycogen storage diseases).

204. Answer is B.

Haemophilia is inherited as a sex-linked disorder.

205. Answer is E.

Red–green colour blindness is inherited as a sex-linked disorder, as is fragile-X and Duchenne muscular dystrophy.

206. Answer is B.

207. Answer is B.

Neurofibromatosis, myotonic dystrophy, and Marfan syndrome are all autosomal dominant.

208. Answer is A.

Smoking cannabis during pregnancy is associated with low birth weight, smaller head circumference, greater risk of miscarriage, especially in those who use marijuana regularly (more than six times per week); these babies, when born, may undergo withdrawal-like symptoms.

Marijuana can reduce fertility in both men and women, making it difficult to conceive in the first place.

However, many women who take illicit drugs also take alcohol and tobacco, and may engage in other unhealthy behaviours, putting their pregnancy at risk; therefore it is difficult to be certain what can be attributed solely to the illicit substances.

209. Answer is E.

210. Answer is A.

211. Answer is C.

212. Answer is D.

213. Answer is F.

214. Answer is A.

Conventional varicose vein surgery is a clinically and cost-effective treatment; laser and radio-frequency treatment replace traditional stripping and most varicosities still need to be treated by sclerotherapy or phlebectomy (*BMJ*, 2006; **333**: 287–92).

215. Answer is B.

Bleeding from a varicosity that has eroded the skin should be referred as an emergency; one which has bled once and is in danger of doing so again should be referred urgently; a progressive, painful ulcer not responding to treatment should be referred quickly, and recurrent superficial thrombophlebitis should be referred as a routine out-patient appointment (*BMJ*, 2006; **333**: 287–92).

216. Answer is A.

Weight gain is a feature of an underactive thyroid.

217. Answer E is false.

Pernicious anaemia leads to a macrocytic anaemia due to vitamin B12 deficiency.

Questions 218–220: See *Br. J. Gen. Pract.* 2013; **63**: 53–4.

218. Answer is A.

219. Answer is B.

220. Answer is B.

221. Answer is C.

Not all women with ectopic pregnancy present with the common symptoms of abdominal / pelvic pain, missed / absent menses, and vaginal bleeding. Other reported symptoms include breast tenderness, gastrointestinal symptoms, dizziness / lightheadedness, shoulder tip pain, urinary symptoms, rectal pressure / pain on defecation. Therefore during clinical assessment of any woman of reproductive age, be aware that they may be pregnant (*NICE CG154*, Dec 2012, *Ectopic pregnancy and miscarriage*).

222. Answer D is true.

Other skin disorders known to koebnerise – that is, the appearance of skin lesions on previously normal skin after an incident of skin injury or trauma include: lichen sclerosis, lichen planus and erythema multiforme.

NICE (July 2006) recommended use of etanercept (a cytokine inhibitor) for the use of severe plaque psoriasis in patients who have not responded to standard systemic treatments.

Tacrolimus is licensed for use in moderate to severe eczema.

223. Answer is D.

Disulfiram is used as an adjunct to treatment of alcohol dependence and gives rise to extremely unpleasant systemic reactions after ingestion of even a small amount of alcohol.

224. Answer is C.

Patients taking monoamine oxidase inhibitors such a moclobemide should not take substances such as Marmite, Bovril, mature cheese, or pickled herring, because of the risk of a dangerous hypertensive crisis.

225. Answer is B.

Grapefruit can increase the risk of rhabdomyolysis as a side-effect of taking simvastatin.

226. Answer is A.

Cranberry juice can raise the INR of patients on warfarin.

227. Answer is C.

When initiating antidepressant treatment in patients with recent myocardial infarction or unstable angina, sertraline is the treatment of choice and has the best evidence base (*NICE CG23*, Dec 2004, April 2007).

There is evidence to show that taking long chain omega-3 fatty acids may help to relieve depression when given in addition to antidepressant therapy, but the evidence is not strong enough to recommend routine supplementation.

228. Answer is D.

(*NICE CG79*, Feb 2009, *Rheumatoid arthritis: the management of rheumatoid arthritis in adults*).

229. Answer is A.

See http://guidance.nice.org.uk/TA/WaveR111/1 [accessed 1 July 2013].

230. Answer is D.

Patient must give consent to inform employer; alternatively, patient may give consent to inform RIDDOR instead; 'industrial' covers all forms of work and is payable even if employee is partially or wholly to blame; effect of injury must persist beyond 91 days to qualify (*Oxford Handbook General Practice*, 2009; see also www.riddor.gov.uk ; www.dwp.gov.uk/healthcare-professional/benefits-and-services/industrial-injuries-disablement/).

231. Answer is A.

232. Answer is D.

233. Answer is E.

234. Answer is C.

235. Answer is B.

236. Answer is F.

237. Answer is B.

238. Answer is G.

239. Answer is H.

240. Answer is I.

241. Answer is D.

242. Answer is E.

243. Answer is D.

Trisomy 21 is also known as Down syndrome.

244. Answer is A.

47XXY is Klinefelter's syndrome.

245. Answer is E.

Trisomy 18 is Edwards' syndrome.

246. Answer is B.

45XO is Turner's syndrome.

247. Answer is F.

Normal genotype for males is 46XY and for females 46XX.

248. Answer is C.

5p deletion (deletion of end of short arm of chromosome 5) results in cri-du-chat syndrome.

249. Answer is D.

Insecticide-treated clothing and insecticide-treated nets are likely to be beneficial; the effectiveness of the others is unknown. There is a consensus that topical insect repellents containing DEET reduce the risk of insect bites, although few studies have been done (*BMJ Clinical Evidence: Malaria – Prevention in Travellers*, October 2006).

250. Answer is B.

Grapefruit juice should be avoided by those on statins.

If antibiotics such as erythromycin or clarithromycin are prescribed, statins should be stopped for that time period.

If a patient is hypertensive and on amlodipine then the simvastatin dose should be limited to 20 mg daily.

Gemfibrozil should not be used with simvastatin; other fibrates can be used but only with a maximum simvastatin dose of 10 mg.

(MHRA Drug and Safety Update 6 (1) 2012; www.wales.nhs.uk/sites3/ Documents/814/SimvastatinAmlodipineInteraction-ABHBfinalSept2012.pdf [accessed 1 July 2013]).

Questions 251–300

for answers see pages 99–104

251. Headache

Which of the following would you use as first-line prophylaxis for a 30 year old male primary school teacher with a clear history of monthly migraine, no red flags and a normal neurological examination?

A Aspirin 900 mg
B Paracetamol 1 g
C Metoclopramide 10 mg
D Propanolol 80 mg
E Almotriptan 12.5 mg
F Combined oral contraceptive pill run consecutively for 2 months at a time

252. Neurology

A 40 year old engineer attends your morning surgery. He awoke that morning and noticed dribbling from the right side of his mouth which was sagging down and he is unable to close his right eye; he is also complaining of ipsilateral sensitivity to loud noises and earache on the same side. When asked to smile, you notice an asymmetry of the mouth.

Which one of the following is untrue?

A When examining him clinically you should check his ears in case he has a rash
B He is presenting with signs of a lower motor lesion of the seventh cranial nerve
C Treating with prednisolone has been shown to significantly improve outcome at 3 and 9 months
D Acyclovir has been shown to add even more significant benefit alone and in combination with prednisolone

253. Rheumatology

A 54 year old woman presents with aching in both hands affecting both thumbs and the first two and a half fingers; symptoms are worse at night when she has to sit up and shake both wrists for relief. You make a diagnosis of carpal tunnel syndrome. The patient would like to discuss treatment options.

Which one of the following has evidence of benefit?

A Diuretics
B Corticosteroid injections
C Nerve and tendon gliding exercises
D Therapeutic ultrasound
E Splints

254–257. Teenage knees

A Chondromalacia patellae
B Osteogenesis imperfecta
C Patellar tendonitis
D Tibial apophysitis
E Osteoarthritis
F Osteochondritis dissecans

Match the following presentations with the single most appropriate diagnosis from the list above.

254. A 15 year old girl gives a 2 month history of anterior knee pain, worse when going up and down stairs and on rising from prolonged sitting.

255. A 14 year old boy gives a 3 month history of pain just below the knee cap. He is getting upset as the pain is always worse after his football sessions; rest alleviates symptoms. On examination you notice a small, tender bony lump a few centimetres below the knee cap.

256. An 18 year old boy who is usually quite athletic has developed pain at the front of his knee; symptoms are worse after running. On examination, the pain is reproduced by resisted knee extension.

257. An 18 year old boy has seen one of your colleagues with knee pain after exercising, associated with intermittent episodes of knee swelling and sometimes locking. You are reviewing his X-ray which shows cartilage damage.

258. Diabetic fitness to drive

Which one of the following is false?
A An insulin-dependent diabetic may drive a Group One vehicle so long as they have no visual impairment and have only hypoglycaemic impairment
B If a patient has a Group Two vehicle licence and has been stable on insulin since 1991, they can continue to drive as long as they have evidence of annual visual checks
C If taking a gliptin, patients do not need to notify the DVLA
D If taking exenatide, patients do not need to notify the DVLA

259–262. Contraception

You are counselling a 22 year old mother of two for contraception. You have duly mentioned LARCs as an option she may wish to consider. She is currently on day 12 of her cycle and her husband, who is in the army, is due home in the next few weeks. She has not been sexually active for the past 3 months and would like to know, if she starts a method of contraception today, how long until it will be effective.

Match the contraceptive with the time frame. Each option may be used once, more than once, or not at all.

A Immediately
B Within 48 hours
C After 7 days

259. Intrauterine device.

260. Medroxyprogesterone acetate injection.

261. Implanon implant.

262. Intrauterine system.

263. Contraindications to IUCD insertion

Which one of the following is not a contraindication to insertion of a copper IUD?

A History of pelvic inflammatory disease when aged 18
B History of ectopic pregnancy
C Known uterine fibroids
D Wilson's disease
E Pregnancy
F Undiagnosed irregular vaginal bleeding

264. Contraindications to the combined oral contraceptive pill

With regard to the combined oral contraceptive pill, which one of the following is not classed as UKMEC4?

A Cervical ectropion
B BMI 42
C Breast cancer
D Migraine with aura
E Personal history of DVT

265–269. Paediatric rashes

Match the clinical scenario to the causative organism

A Rubella
B Herpes virus HSV6
C Chicken pox virus
D Coxsackie virus
E Parvovirus B19
F Measles

265. A 7 year boy attends having had a fever and raised facial erythema; the nasolabial folds and circum-oral region were spared but now, 2 days later, he has a lacy erythema affecting the extremities and going up towards the buttocks.

266. A 4 year old boy has been complaining of a painful back for the past few days. He was seen by one of your colleagues 2 days ago who advised his mother to bring the child back if symptoms persisted. On examination there is red plaque running from the left side of the vertebral column around to the axilla in a longitudinal pattern; the child will not let you touch the area which is covered in small clear vesicles.

267. An 18 month old child has had a high fever; this came down this morning but the parents have noted a rash. There are pink, almond-shaped macules on the trunk, but the child is well, compared to previously.

268. A 4 year old child is brought in having been sent home from school; mum is very flustered as it is the first day back after the Easter break. The child is complaining of a sore painful mouth, is refusing to eat and has a high fever. On examination, you notice multiple aphthous ulcers and, on removing the child's socks, you notice two small macular lesions. There are no lesions anywhere else.

269. You see a miserable 5 year old child whose mother owns the local health food shop; she is worried that her daughter has been unwell for the past 3 days with a fever, malaise, runny nose, and what she has been treating as conjunctivitis. On examination of the ears, nose and throat you notice a rash behind the ears and blue–white spots on a red background on the buccal mucosa opposite the upper premolar teeth.

270. Low back pain

For which one of the following causes of low back pain is X-ray of the lumbar spine routinely indicated?

A Spinal malignancy
B Infection
C Fracture
D Cauda equina syndrome
E Ankylosing spondylitis
F All of the above
G None of the above.

271. Low back pain

Which one of the following treatment options should not be offered in the treatment of persistent non-specific low back pain?

A Strong opioids
B Simple paracetamol
C Acupuncture
D Tricyclic antidepressants
E Injection of therapeutic substances

272–277. Ophthalmology

A Chlamydial conjunctivitis
B Allergic conjunctivitis
C Bacterial conjunctivitis
D Acute iritis
E Scleritis
F Ophthalmia neonatorum

For each of the scenarios given below, which one of the above is the single most likely diagnosis?

272. A 47 year old man with a long history of back pain, psoriasis, and known to be HLAB27-positive, presents with severe pain and redness affecting one eye.

273. An 8 year old child presents with irritation of the right eye and difficulty opening his eyes in the morning due to a sticky discharge.

274. A 24 year old mother attends with bilateral irritation, itching and watering of the eyes; on everting the tarsal plate you note large papillae.

275. An 18 year old student has had conjunctivitis for more than 2 weeks now; he is otherwise fit and well but is getting upset at the redness of his eyes and persistent mucopurulent discharge; he denies any other symptoms.

276. Your 38 year old receptionist asks you to look at her eye which suddenly became painful earlier in the morning. Shining a light into the eye is painful for her and you notice that her pupil is irregularly shaped. She has had this problem a number of times in the past but has run out of the drops she was given by the specialist to use if the symptoms recurred.

277. A 2 week old baby is brought in with bilateral sticky eyes and a heavy conjunctival discharge. Mum thought it was sticky eye, but on examination you note both conjunctivae are infected and the upper eyelids are slightly puffy and red.

278–283. Evidence-based medicine

A   Cohort study
B   Case-control study
C   Meta-analysis
D   Cross-sectional survey
E   Case report
F   Randomised controlled trials
G   CONSORT

Match the description below with one type of study listed above.

278. A descriptive snap-shot that looks at the prevalence of a particular disease or condition; it cannot be used to calculate the incidence.

279. A retrospective study which cannot calculate the incidence nor prove causation, but can be used to calculate the odds ratio.

280. A prospective, observational study that can be used to calculate the incidence of a disease and its relative risk.

281. This describes the medical history of a single patient in the form of a narrative.

282. The recommended format for reporting randomised controlled trials in medical journals.

283. Considered to be the best way to compare the effectiveness of different interventions; allows valid inferences of cause and effect.

284–289. Evidence-based medicine

Place the study types below in order of hierarchy of evidence, starting with (for question 284) the study design that carries most weight, and ending (for question 289) with the study design that carries the least weight.

A   Cohort study
B   Case-control study
C   Meta-analysis
D   Cross-sectional survey
E   Case report
F   Randomised controlled trials

290. Odds ratio

Treatment	Total number of patients treated	Number whose symptoms resolved within 24 hours	Number whose symptoms did not resolve within 24 hours
Drug X	50	40	10
Placebo	50	20	30

Select the correct odds ratio from the list below:
A   2
B   4
C   6
D   8

291. Neonatal jaundice

You are asked at the end of your morning surgery to pay a house call to visit a mother who recently gave birth; she was discharged from hospital at 10 am having had an uneventful delivery at 3 am. Mum has noticed that the baby looks a funny colour and would like your advice as to what to do. Mum has decided she will breast feed. When you examine the baby, you note that he has yellow sclera and is jaundiced.

What should you do?
A   Refer immediately back to hospital to exclude infection and/or haemolysis
B   Reassure mum that this is very common in breast-fed babies and should clear in due course
C   Advise mum to put the baby in direct sunlight
D   Await result of Guthrie test in 6 days as jaundice may be due to hypothyroidism

292. Health and safety regulations in general practice

Which one of the following statements is untrue?
A   Arrangements for the disposal of clinical waste should comply with health and safety regulations and the requirements of the Environmental Protection Act 1990
B   Only premises with 10 employees or more are required by law to have a written safety policy
C   An employer has the option of either displaying the official poster setting out the law or issuing employees with the corresponding leaflet
D   An employer is required to consult with employees about health and safety arrangements and their implementation

293–295. Acute paediatrics

A IM benzyl penicillin 300 mg
B IM benzyl penicillin 600 mg
C IM benzyl penicillin 1.2 g

In the case of a child presenting with headache, photophobia, neck stiffness, impaired levels of consciousness, and a non-blanching haemorrhagic rash, match the dose and route of administration of penicillin to the age group.

293. Age 12 months

294. Age 6 years

295. Age 11 years

296–298. Asthma

A Double the dose of the inhaled corticosteroid
B Try a long-acting beta-2 agonist
C Try a short-acting muscarinic antagonist
D Consider addition of a leukotriene receptor antagonist
E Refer to a respiratory specialist
F Continue as is for now

For each of the scenarios given below, which one of the above would you do next?

296. Tom is 4 years old and attends surgery with mum who is worried about his cough. Despite taking regular standard dose inhaled corticosteroid as beclomethasone dipropionate twice daily he is still experiencing cough, wheeze and needing to use his short-acting beta agonist four times a day. Mum reports he responds quickly to his reliever but isn't sure how often he should be taking it.

You check the technique of inhaler use, which is good and examine the respiratory tract, which is normal.

297. Tom's brother Gareth is the next patient and is two years older.

He presents in the same way as Tom in that he has persistent cough, wheeze and despite taking beclomethasone dipropionate 100 mcg bd is finding his asthma is not controlled.

298. The last patient of the morning's surgery is Tina, Tom and Gareth's mum.

At her last visit you agreed that her previous regime of a short-acting beta agonist and standard dose beclomethasone dipropionate at 200 mcg bd was not controlling her asthma, so you prescribed a long-acting beta-agonist to help.

She is happy to report that having been on it for two weeks she feels much better and would like to know what to do next.

299. Blindness

Which one of the following statements is true?
A Partial sightedness implies vision < 3/60
B Blindness is defined as the inability to perform any work for which eye sight is essential
C Blindness is defined as the total absence of sight
D When considering Registration of blindness, most people who are eligible are registered
E Registration of blindness does not make a difference to a person's tax allowance or benefits

300. Diabetic neuropathic pain

You see a 64 year old lady who has had type 2 diabetes for the past 20 years; she complains bitterly of shooting pains in both lower limbs and numbness in her toes.

After examining her you make a diagnosis of diabetic neuropathic pain.

What is the first line medication you would offer?

....

Answers to questions 251–300

251. Answer is D.

SIGN guidelines (107, 2008) state that beta blockers should be used as first-line prophylaxis. The other options, excluding F, are useful for treatment of acute episodes, with metoclopramide being particularly helpful for patients with nausea and vomiting. Option F is a red herring and a reminder to read each question carefully.

> Note that management of common neurological conditions such as tension headache and migraine have been identified as areas causing difficulty for candidates sitting recent AKTs.

252. Answer is D.

This man has Bell's palsy, a seventh cranial nerve palsy. In upper motor lesions the eye is unaffected in which case one should be thinking of stroke. Ear examination is performed to look for a vesicular rash (Ramsay–Hunt Syndrome from varicella zoster – seen in approximately 50% of cases).

An RCT in *NEJM* (2007; **357**: 1598–1607) concluded that prednisolone significantly improved outcomes at 3 months (NNT = 6) and 9 months (NNT = 8), but that acyclovir did not.

Suggest 25 mg bd for 10/7 within 72 hours of the onset of symptoms.

253. Answer is B.

Clinical Evidence (June 2007) showed only steroid injections as having evidence of effectiveness; the other options were deemed unlikely to be beneficial; NSAIDs were classed as being of unknown effectiveness.
With regard to management of carpal tunnel syndrome, in mild cases, initial treatment should include the use of wrist splints. If this fails, then a local corticosteroid injection is appropriate, but it is not clear what the best regimen is to use. Patients with severe or persistent impairment, or symptoms that do not respond to splinting or an injection, should be referred for consideration of decompression surgery (*Drug and Therapeutics Bulletin*, 2009; **47**: 86–89).

254. Answer is A.

This is very common in teenage girls. Advise analgesia and physiotherapy including vastus medialis strengthening which has been shown to relieve pain in 80% cases (*Oxford Handbook of General Practice*, 2005).

255. Answer is D.

Also known as Osgood–Schlatter disease. This is, again, very common in sporty teenagers, especially boys engaged in a lot of kicking; not so common over the age of 16. Simple painkillers and rest will suffice in most cases, but refer if symptoms persist.

256. Answer is C.

Could be confused with Osgood–Schlatter disease, but the clue is in the clinical examination. Rest, NSAIDs and consider steroid injection around tendon.

257. Answer is E.

Pain is due to necrosis of the articular cartilage and underlying bone. Seen in young adults, it can predispose to OA so suggest referral on to specialist care.

258. Answer is B.

Group One vehicles include cars and motorcycles; Group Two vehicles include lorries and buses.

In the case of an insulin-dependent diabetic, if the Group Two licence was issued after 1991, then it is revoked. Any cases where the licence was issued before 1/4/1991 are considered by the DVLA on a case by case basis.

259. Answer is A.

260. Answer is C.

261. Answer is C.

262. Answer is C.

NICE (*Long Acting Reversible Contraception: CG30,* Oct 2005) states that LARC methods are more cost-effective than the combined oral contraceptive pill even at 1 year of use. Of these, IUDs, the IUS and the implant are more cost-effective than injectable contraceptives.

263. Answer is A.

An IUD should not be inserted if the patient has a history of PID or has been exposed to a sexually transmitted disease, although it may be inserted 3 months after infection if there are no signs of persisting infection; always swab first (World Health Organization; *Medical eligibility criteria for contraceptive use: WHOMEC 3rd edition*).

264. Answer is A.

The UK Medical Eligibility Criteria (UKMEC) are a set of evidence-based recommendations designed to help women select the most appropriate method of contraception for specific clinical conditions without imposing unnecessary restrictions (Faculty of Family Planning and Reproductive Health Care: *UK medical eligibility criteria for contraceptive use* (2006); www.ffprhc.org.uk [accessed 1 July 2013]).

UKMEC4 are considered to be conditions where to prescribe the COCP would pose an unacceptable health risk, i.e. an absolute contraindication. UKMEC1 are conditions where there is no restriction on the use of the contraceptive method with UKMEC3 and UKMEC2 lying in between.

> Note that feedback from previous AKTs has identified contraindications to oral contraceptives and to IUCD as areas of weakness amongst candidates.

265. Answer is E.

This is erythema infectiosum, also known as Fifth disease. The facial rash will fade within a few days and the rash on the legs within a few weeks.

266. Answer is C.

This reactivation of chicken pox virus is herpes zoster. It usually occurs in a single dermatome and, classically, the rash does not cross the midline.

267. Answer is B.

This is roseola infantum; the rash can last up to 2 days.

268. Answer is D.

This is hand, foot and mouth disease which is more common in spring. The macular rash on the hands and/or feet often goes on to blister; the lesions last 3-5 days and heal without scarring.

269. Answer is F.

This is measles. The spots inside the mouth are Koplik's spots and are pathognomonic for this disease.

270. Answer is G.

NICE Guideline CG88: Low back pain: early management of persistent non-specific low back pain (May 2009) suggests that for these conditions an MRI should be considered.

271. Answer is E.

NICE Guideline CG88 advises against offering injections of therapeutic substances into the back for non-specific low back pain; strong opioids can be used for short-term use in people with severe pain.

272. Answer is D.

Try NSAID; may need systemic steroids.

273. Answer is C.

Try topical antibiotic.

274. Answer is B.

Try topical antihistamine.

275. Answer is A.

Refer for testing and contact tracing.

276. Answer is E.

Use topical steroids and arrange ophthalmology review.

277. Answer is F.

A notifiable disease; refer immediately for testing and treatment; will need to examine mum too.

278. Answer is D.

279. Answer is B.

280. Answer is A.

281. Answer is E.

For example: "Mrs M is a forty one year old woman presenting with lower abdominal pain...".

282. Answer is G.

The new CONSORT statement lists 21 items that should be included in a report as well as a flow chart describing patient progress through the trial. In the spirit of the times, the recommendations are evidence-based where possible, with common sense dictating the remainder. The CONSORT statement means that authors will no longer be able to hide inadequacies in their study by omitting important information. For example, authors cannot hide their procedures behind the single word "randomised", they must give details of the randomisation procedure (*BMJ*, 1996, **313**: 570–571).

283. Answer is F.

284. Answer is C.

285. Answer is F.

286. Answer is A.

287. Answer is B.

288. Answer is D.

289. Answer is E.

These answers assume all else is equal; obviously a heavily biased, poorly randomised RCT will carry less weight than a well designed cohort study.

290. Answer is C.

The odds ratio is a way of comparing whether the probability of a certain event is the same for two groups. It is calculated by dividing the experimental events odds (40/10) by the control events odds (20/30), as follows:

40/10 = 4

20/30 = 2/3

4 divided by 2/3 is the same as 4 multiplied by 3/2 = 12/2 = 6.

 Note that in recent feedback on candidates' performance in the AKT, the RCGP has flagged EBM as an area causing difficulty for candidates and specific mention has been made of the odds ratio.

291. Answer is A.

Any jaundice in the first 24 hours is assumed to be pathological and needs immediate hospital referral; the child may need antibiotics, phototherapy or exchange transfusion.

292. Answer is B.

Premises with five or more employees are required by law to have a written safety policy (*Health and Safety in General Practice: a guide to risk assessment for GPs and practice managers;* www.gserve.nice.org.uk/nicemedia/ documents/has_riskassgps.pdf [accessed 1 July 2013]).

Note that the RCGP has specifically mentioned risk management and health and safety as areas where candidates have difficulty and therefore areas they plan to continue testing in.

293. Answer is A.

294. Answer is B.

295. Answer is C.

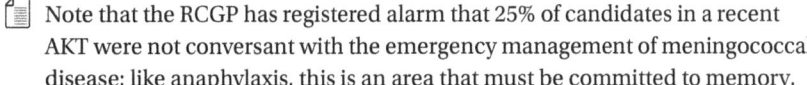 Note that the RCGP has registered alarm that 25% of candidates in a recent AKT were not conversant with the emergency management of meningococcal disease; like anaphylaxis, this is an area that must be committed to memory.

Questions 296–298: See www.brit-thoracic.org.uk/Portals/0/ Guidelines/AsthmaGuidelines/qrg101%202011.pdf [accessed 1 July 2013].

The British Thoracic Society Guideline on the Management of Asthma was revised in January 2012 and sets out in detail the management of asthma in adults and children, which differs in certain important areas.

296. Answer is D.

297. Answer is B.

298. Answer is F.

If the patient has a good response to the LABA then this should be continued.

299. Answer is B.

Oxford Handbook of General Practice, 2nd edition (2005).

Although sick certification is a daily task of general practice, rules governing other types of certification and registration, such as those for blindness, should also be known.

300. Answer is duloxetine (usual starting dose 60 mg/day, maximum 120 mg/day).

(*NICE CG96*, March 2010, *Neuropathic pain: the pharmacological management of neuropathic pain in adults in non-specialist settings*).

Recent AKT papers have included this type of fill in the blank question.

Questions 301-350

for answers see pages 113–118

301. Mental health

A 40 year old man recently started on lithium would experience which of the following side-effects if he developed lithium toxicity?

A Weight gain
B Dry mouth
C Altered taste sensation
D Mild nausea
E Coarse tremor

302-304. Practice admin

A purple
B red
C yellow

Match the booklet to the patient held record:

302. Lithium.

303. Child health surveillance.

304. Warfarin.

305. Anticoagulation

Your practice nurse is away and you are asked to call patients with their INRs and advise them on their warfarin dose. You call an elderly lady whose INR is 1.8; notes show that her AF requires this to be between 2 and 3. When you call to advise her to increase her dose she tells you she is currently taking a blue one, a pink one and a brown one.

How much warfarin is this lady taking?

A 5 mg
B 6 mg
C 7 mg
D 8 mg

306. Depression

A 52 year old lady presents with moderate depression after a diagnosis of breast cancer; she has been put on tamoxifen by her specialist. She has been referred for CBT but her therapist feels she would benefit from an antidepressant.

Which one of the following would be the best antidepressant for her?
A Paroxetine
B Fluoxetine
C Sertraline
D Duloxetine
E Citalopram

307. Travel-related venous thromboembolism

You are consulted by a 54 year old woman who is usually fit and well with no past medical history. She is planning on flying to Egypt from the UK in a few weeks but is worried as her BMI is 30 and she has heard of the risks of blood clots when travelling.

Which one of the following would you advise her to do?
A Take regular walks and do calf stretches during the flight
B Take a low dose (75 mg) aspirin thirty minutes before flying and again four hours later
C Purchase grade 2 below-knee compression stockings for her and her partner
D Refrain from all alcohol during the flight
E Request upgrade to business class on basis of health

308. Fit notes

You see a patient who has already submitted a self-certificate for one week. You feel they would benefit from another week off work; *how many statements of fitness to work (sick notes) do you issue at this review appointment?*
A 1
B 2
C 2, but write 'Duplicate' on the second
D None – they are allowed to self-certify for another week if it is the same illness

309-312. Genetics

A 30 year old man attends with his wife for results of semen analysis prior to an infertility referral. She has had routine blood tests which confirm she is ovulating; you note he is tall at 189 cm, has narrow shoulders, wide hips, sparse facial hair.

His semen analysis is well below normal and you wonder if he may have Klinefelter's syndrome.

Fill in the following table with the correct frequencies of clinical conditions associated with this syndrome.
A   3%
B   10%
C   20%
D   40%

309. Metabolic syndrome

310. Breast cancer

311. Type 2 diabetes mellitus

312. Osteoporosis

313. Atrial fibrillation

You note Mr Elliot, 76 years old and otherwise fit and well, to be in AF at a rate of 92 bpm. He has no other health issues.

Which one of the following is correct?
A   His CHADS$_2$ score is 1 so he does not need warfarin
B   His CHADS$_2$ score is 1 but his age means he should be offered warfarin
C   Rate control is the most appropriate in this case
D   Digoxin is still the first-line rate control agent with beta blockers or rate-limiting calcium antagonists as second line

314. Screening of the newborn

The NHS Newborn Blood Spot Screening Programme offers screening for all of the following conditions except which one?
A   Phenylketonuria
B   Congenital hypothyroidism
C   Medium-chain acyl-CoA dehydrogenase deficiency
D   Thalassaemia
E   Cystic fibrosis

315. Diabetic eye screening in adults

Which one of the following statements is incorrect?

A Diabetic eye screening is offered annually to people with diabetes from the age of 12

B The aim of the programme is to reduce the risk of sight loss among people with diabetes, by the prompt identification and effective treatment if necessary of sight-threatening diabetic retinopathy, at the appropriate stage during the disease process

C In pregnancy women with type 1 diabetes are offered a diabetic retinopathy screen when they first present for care

D In pregnancy women with type 2 diabetes are not offered a diabetic retinopathy screen when they first present for care, as they are at much lower risk

316–321. Screening in adults

A Prostate screening
B Diabetic eye screening
C Bowel cancer screening
D Breast screening
E Cervical screening
F Abdominal aortic aneurysm screening

For each patient group detailed below, select the single most appropriate screening option from the list above. Each stem may be used once, more than once, or not at all.

316. All men in their 65th year; men older than this can self-refer

317. Men and women aged 60–69, every two years; those aged 70 or over can be tested on request

318. Women aged 50–70, every three years

319. A woman aged over 70 can self-refer for this, but will not automatically be called

320. Women aged 25–49, every three years

321. Women aged 50–64, every five years

322. Calculating drug doses

Baby Sebastian has just been discharged from hospital and the discharge summary states that he requires azithromycin 80 mg three times weekly through his enteral feeding tube; the suspension comes as 200 mg in 5 ml.

Mum would like to know how much she should give. *What would you advise her?*

A 1 ml
B 2 ml
C 3 ml
D 4 ml
E 5 ml

323. LARC implants

A 41 year old lady presents on day four of her menstrual cycle to have an implant fitted; she had a baby four months previously.

Which one of the following is true?

A You should advise her that she may have the implant fitted that day but needs to use additional contraceptive precautions, such as a barrier method, for the next seven days
B No routine follow-up is needed unless she has problems
C Mifepristone is effective at controlling irregular bleeding associated with implant and is licensed for this indication
D Due to her age, this lady may be better suited to DMPA injection

324. Controlled drugs

You are issued with a drugs box by your practice on the first day you join them. It includes two ampoules of morphine for injection which you have been asked to 'sign for'.

Which one of the following statements is untrue regarding Schedule 2 controlled drugs (CDs)?

A They must be stored in a locked receptacle, usually in an appropriate CD cabinet or approved safe, which can only be opened by the person in lawful possession of the CD or a person authorised by that person
B Where a practitioner carries a bag for home visits it is acceptable for them to be in a locked bag in a locked boot
C Validity of any prescription for Schedule 2 CDs is restricted to 24 days
D CD prescriptions can be typewritten, handwritten or computer printed
E A register must be kept for Schedule 2 CDs
F There is no current legal requirement that 'patient-returned' Schedule 2 CDs should be destroyed in the presence of an authorised witness

325. Osteoporosis

Which one of the following is true about osteoporosis?

A   All men and women aged 65 years and over should be considered for assessment of fracture risk

B   People under the age of 50 should not be routinely assessed as they are thought to be at low risk

C   Risk assessment tools, such as FRAX or QFracture, can reliably be used to estimate risk in people with alcoholism

D   Proton pump inhibitors do not affect fracture risk

E   Selective serotonin reuptake inhibitors do not affect fracture risk

326-336. Developmental milestones

A   Age 1
B   Age 2
C   Age 3
D   Age 4
E   Age 5

Match the milestone to the age by which most children have achieved it.

326. Stands independently

327. Copies a vertical line

328. Jumps

329. Copies a cross

330. Can speak a two word sentence, e.g. 'want drink'

331. Skips

332. Drinks from a cup using two hands

333. Is able to wave bye-bye

334. Can build a tower of four or more blocks

335. Can build a tower of six or more blocks

336. Is able to pour, cut with supervision, and mash own food

337. Developmental delay

The parents of the following children present concerned about developmental delay. *In which scenario would you be least inclined to refer for assessment of developmental delay?*

A   A child who is unable to sit unsupported by 9 months
B   A child who is not walking by 18 months
C   A child who has not been seen to fix and follow at 3 months
D   A ten month old who is still using exclusively a palmar grasp
E   A child whose parents have noted a preference to use the left hand at nine months

338-343. Qualitative studies

In the *British Journal of General Practice* (December 2012) I read an article entitled:

'Integrating online communities and social networks with computerised treatment for insomnia.'

The following are extracts from the method, results and discussion part of the paper; *please fill in the blanks using the options given below.*

Method: **338**.......... semi-structured interviews and **339**.......... were used to capture a breadth and depth of perspectives from service users with sleep problems and a range of health professionals, **340**......... recruited from Lincolnshire and Nottinghamshire, UK.

Results: Two **341**.......... emerged from the data: trust and functionality.

Discussion: The strengths of this study were an exploration by a multidisciplinary team of different perspectives, **342**.......... of data and **343**.......... from a wide range of patients and health professionals.

A   qualitative
B   purposively
C   themes
D   focus groups
E   triangulation
F   divergent case analysis

344. Conception and fertility

A couple do not use contraception, have regular sexual intercourse and the woman is under 40 years of age. *What is the percentage chance of them conceiving within one year?*

A   80%
B   70%
C   60%
D   50%

345. Fertility

Which one of the following is true?

A   Men with a BMI over 30 should be reassured that they are unlikely to have impaired fertility

B   The recommended dose of folic acid for women who have diabetes is 400 mcg

C   A woman with a 34 day menstrual cycle should have a blood test to check for serum progesterone levels in the mid-luteal phase of her menstrual cycle to confirm ovulation on day 27

D   The use of basal body temperature charts to confirm ovulation is highly predictive and is recommended

E   Prolactin levels, thyroid functions tests, follicle-stimulating hormones and luteinising hormone should be checked in women concerned about their fertility

346. Steroids

Which of the following is the weakest steroid?

A   Clobetasone (Eumovate, Trimovate plus oxytetracycline and nystatin)

B   Clobetasol (Dermovate)

C   Hydrocortisone acetate (hydrocortisone strength ≤2.5%)

D   Hydrocortisone butyrate (0.1%) (locoid)

347-350. Fingertip units

A   One
B   Two
C   Three
D   Four

Match the fingertip units to the dose or skin area to be covered when using steroids for eczema. Each stem may be used once, more than once, or not at all.

347. 1 g of steroid

348. 4 month old baby's trunk

349. one adult hand

350. 4 year old child's trunk

Answers to questions 301-350

---

301. Answer is E.

Coarse tremor is a sign of lithium toxicity and warrants immediate review of the patient, urgent bloods and possible admission (*BMJ*, 2010; **341:** c6258).

Expected side-effects of lithium	Key features of lithium toxicity
• Fine tremor • Dry mouth • Altered taste sensation • Increased thirst • Increased frequency of urination • Mild nausea • Weight gain	• Vomiting or diarrhoea • Coarse tremor (larger movements, especially of hands) • Muscle weakness • General lack of coordination, including ataxia • Slurred speech • Blurred vision • Lethargy • Confusion • Seizures

Questions 302–304: These are worth looking at whenever your patients come in.

302. Answer is A.

303. Answer is B.

304. Answer is C.

305. Answer is D.

Warfarin comes in a range of colours and strengths. In the UK, the strengths and colours of tablets are as follows:
- 1 mg – brown tablets
- 3 mg – blue tablets
- 5 mg – pink tablets

306. Answer is E.

A number of studies have looked at the interaction between antidepressants, some of which have the ability to inhibit CYP2D6 (the enzyme that converts tamoxifen to its active form endoxifen), and tamoxifen.

They have found that certain ones (e.g. venlafaxine) had a minimal interaction while others, such as paroxetine and fluoxetine, had a very strong interaction and could therefore reduce the effect of tamoxifen in women with breast cancer.

(*BMJ*, 2010, **340:** c783; *BMJ*, 2010, **340:** c693; www.ncbi.nlm.nih.gov/pubmed/20156115 [accessed 1 July 2013]).

307. Answer is A.

Although developing a travel-related DVT/VTE is unlikely in most cases, several factors may increase an individual's risk of developing a DVT/VTE on long-distance flights. These include previous DVT/VTE or known thrombophilic disorder; malignancy; recent (within four weeks) surgery or trauma; immobility; oestrogen use or pregnancy; and sitting in a window seat.

For travellers with an increased risk for travel-related DVT/VTE, the guidelines recommend frequent ambulation, calf muscle stretching, sitting in an aisle seat if possible, or the use of below-knee graduated compression stockings – class 1 are usually sufficient.

There is no definitive evidence to support the belief that dehydration, alcohol intake or sitting in economy class increase a patient's risk for developing a DVT/VTE resulting from long-distance flights.

(www.sign.ac.uk/pdf/qrg122.pdf; www.bcshguidelines.com/documents/BCSHTravelGuidelineFinal190910_(2).pdf; www.cks.nhs.uk/dvt_prevention_for_travellers; www.nhs.uk/news/2012/02February/Pages/economy-class-syndrome-dvt-myth.aspx [all accessed 1 July 2013]).

308. Answer is A.

You can only issue a duplicate Med 3 if the original statement has been lost. You should clearly mark it 'Duplicate'.

Advise people with more than one employer to submit the statement to their main employer, who can note the details of the advice you have given. They can then present the statement to their second employer.

(www.dwp.gov.uk/healthcare-professional/news/statement-of-fitness-for-work.shtml [accessed 1 July 2013]).

Questions 309–312: When seeing a man with this condition you should consider screening tests for diabetes, dyslipidaemia and osteoporosis (*BMJ*, 2012, **345:** e7558).

309. Answer is D.

310. Answer is A.

311. Answer is C.

312. Answer is B.

313. Answer B is correct.

His $CHADS_2$ score is 1:

Risk factor	Score
Congestive cardiac failure	1
Hypertension	1
Age 75 or more	1
Diabetes	1
Stroke or TIA history	2

But it is his age that warrants that he be offered warfarin; rhythm control is more appropriate for those aged less than 65.

Digoxin has been replaced as the first-line rate control agent by beta blockers or rate-limiting calcium channel antagonists such as diltiazem or verapamil (*NICE Guidance CG36* (2006)).

314. Answer is C.

MCADD stands for medium-chain acyl-coenzyme A dehydrogenase deficiency.

315. Answer D is incorrect.

All women who have existing diabetes are offered diabetic eye screening annually; in pregnancy they are also offered it when they first present for care.

Questions 316–321: The RCGP has commented on candidates' lack of knowledge of screening programmes and stated that this area will be tested in every AKT, so it is worth visiting www.screening.nhs.uk.

316. Answer is F.

317. Answer is C.

318. Answer is D.

319. Answer is D.

320. Answer is E.

321. Answer is E.

322. Answer is B.

There are 200 mg in 5 ml; therefore there are 40 mg in 1 ml and 80 mg in 2ml.

Over the last few papers, questions requiring simple calculations of doses of medications have started to appear, but the RCGP has commented that it feels there is still room for improvement.

323. Answer B is true.

Extra precautions are not needed unless it is more than five days since menstrual bleeding started; mifepristone is effective but is not licensed for this indication.

NICE Guidance CG30 (March 2005, updated April 2013) *Long-acting reversible contraception* states that 'irregular bleeding associated with implant use can be treated with mefenamic acid or ethinylestradiol.'

Over the age of 40 there are no specific restrictions on the use of IUS, IUD or implants but with DMPA the risks are thought to outweigh the benefits.

(http://publications.nice.org.uk/long-acting-reversible-contraception-cg30 [accessed 1 July 2013]).

The RCGP has noted this as an area where candidates need to improve their knowledge.

324. Answer C is untrue.

Validity of any prescription for Schedule 2 CDs is in fact 28 days (www.legislation.gov.uk/uksi/2006/3148/contents/made; *Safer management of controlled drugs: early action* (Department of Health, 2007); *Safer management of controlled drugs: guidance on Standard Operating Procedures for controlled drugs* (Department of Health, 2007) [accessed 1 July 2013].

The RCGP has stated that 'although controlled drugs may only infrequently be kept by practices or by GPs in emergency bags, candidates should be familiar with regulations related to prescribing, storage, disposal and register requirements.'

325. Answer B is true.

Women over the age of 65 and men over the age of 75 should be assessed.

Other drugs that may impair bone metabolism include anticonvulsants, selective serotonin reuptake inhibitors, thiazolidinediones, proton pump inhibitors and antiretroviral drugs.

(http://publications.nice.org.uk/osteoporosis-assessing-the-risk-of-fragility-fracture-cg146/guidance [accessed 1 July 2013]).

The RCGP has noted that candidates seem unfamiliar with areas concerning the diagnosis of osteoporosis; NICE has issued recent guidelines (August 2012), the subject appeared in QOF for the first time in 2012/13 and there was also an article in the *BJGP* in December 2012 discussing the guideline's main points.

326. Answer is A.

327. Answer is C.

328. Answer is C.

329. Answer is D.

330. Answer is B.

331. Answer is E.

332. Answer is A.

333. Answer is A.

334. Answer is B.

335. Answer is C.

336. Answer is D.

337. Answer is D.

Most children are able to use a pincer grip by between 9 and 10 months; failure to do so by 12 months, however, should cause concern, as should failure to sit at 9 months, walk by 18 months, fix and follow at 3 months and show hand dominance before one year.

Developmental milestones are an area that is tested regularly; I found it easiest to learn the milestones by spending time with my friends' children as this gave me a better feel for 'what was normal'.

Questions 338–343: Answers drawn from *BJGP*, 2012, **62:** e840–e850(11).

338. Answer is A.

339. Answer is D.

340. Answer is B.

341. Answer is C.

342. Answer is E.

343. Answer is F.

344. Answer is A.

Therefore a woman of reproductive age who has not conceived after one year of unprotected vaginal sexual intercourse, in the absence of any known cause for infertility, should be offered further clinical assessment and investigation along with her partner.

345. Answer C is true.

Both men and women with high BMIs are likely to have reduced fertility.

The dose of folic acid for women with diabetes is 5 mg as they are at increased risk of neural tube defects.

Prolactin levels should only be done in women who have an ovulatory disorder, galactorrhoea or a pituitary tumour.

Women with infertility are no more likely than the general population to have thyroid disease, so do not offer tests for this routinely.

For more information see *NICE CG156* (February 2013), *Fertility* (http://guidance.nice.org.uk/CG156/NICEGuidance/pdf/English [accessed 1 July 2013]).

346. Answer is C.

See *BNF 65* (March 2013).

347. Answer is B.

348. Answer is A.

349. Answer is A.

350. Answer is C.

Algorithm questions 1-77

for answers see pages 131–141

1-8. Medical management of osteoporosis

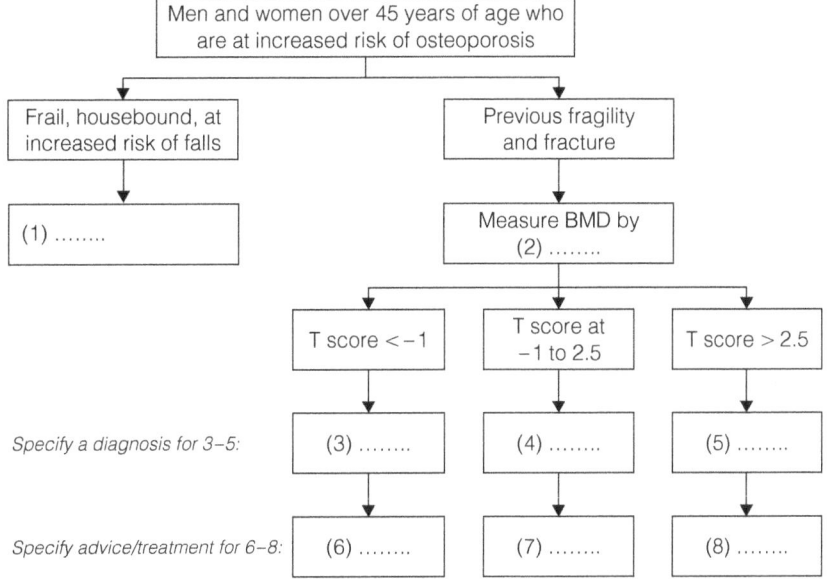

For each of the numbered gaps above, select one option from the list below to complete the algorithm, based on current evidence.

A   Calcium plus vit D supplements; falls assessment and advice; hip protectors

B   Dual Energy X-ray Absorptionometry

C   CT scan

D   MRI scan

E   Normal

F   Osteopenia

G   Osteoporosis

H   Osteomalacia

I   Rickets

J   Reassure; lifestyle advice (nutrition, vitamin D, Ca); regular weight-bearing exercise; reduce smoking; reduce alcohol

K   Lifestyle advice and treat if previous fracture

L   Lifestyle advice and offer treatment

9-12. Medical management of actinic keratoses

```
                        ┌──────────────────────┐
                        │  Actinic keratoses   │
                        └──────────────────────┘
        ┌───────────────────────┼───────────────────────┐
        ▼                       ▼                       ▼
┌─────────────────┐   ┌─────────────────┐   ┌─────────────────┐
│   History of    │   │     Single      │   │    Multiple     │
│  rapid growth   │   │     lesion      │   │     lesions     │
└─────────────────┘   └─────────────────┘   └─────────────────┘
        ▼                       ▼                       │
┌─────────────────┐   ┌─────────────────┐               │
│   (9) ........  │   │   (10) ........ │               │
│                 │   │  if available, or│              │
└─────────────────┘   └─────────────────┘               ▼
                              ▼             ┌─────────────────┐
                      ┌─────────────────┐   │   (11) ........ │
                      │   (11) ........ │   │                 │
                      │ if (10) not available│             │
                      └─────────────────┘   └─────────────────┘
                              ▼
                      ┌─────────────────┐
                      │  Side-effects   │
                      │    tolerated    │
                      └─────────────────┘
              ┌───────────────┴───────────────┐
              ▼                               ▼
      ┌───────────────┐               ┌───────────────┐
      │     Yes       │               │      No       │
      └───────────────┘               └───────────────┘
              ▼                               ▼
      ┌───────────────┐               ┌───────────────┐
      │  Keep under   │ ◄──────────── │  (12) ........ │
      │    review     │               │               │
      └───────────────┘               └───────────────┘
```

For each of the numbered gaps above, select one option from the list below to complete the algorithm, based on current evidence.

A   3% diclofenac cream

B   10% diclofenac cream

C   Cryotherapy

D   Urgent referral

E   5% fluorouracil cream

13-19. Medical management of a patient with atrial fibrillation

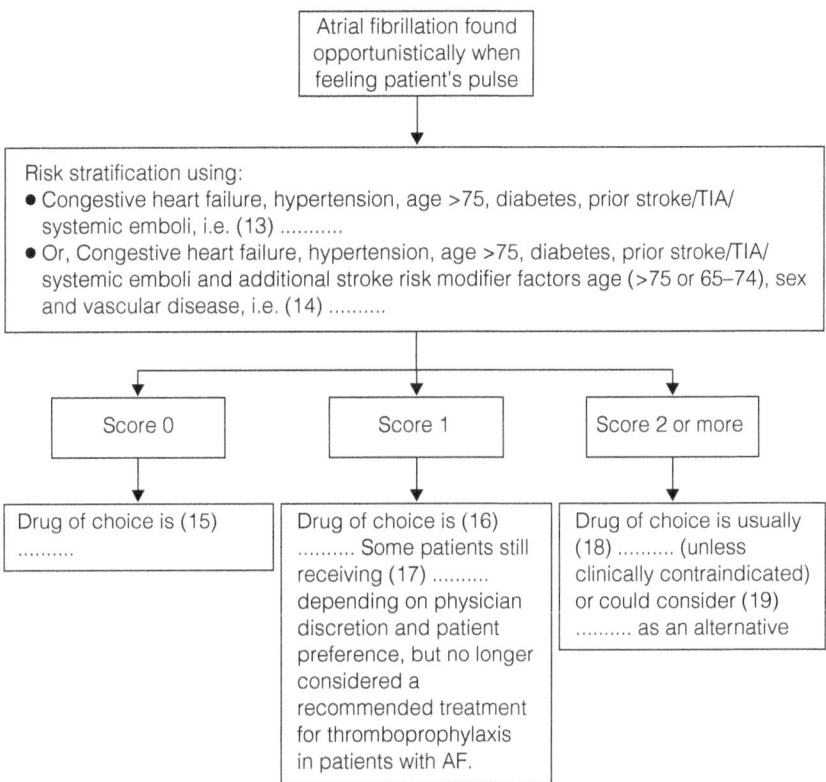

For each of the numbered gaps above, select one option from the list below to complete the algorithm based on current evidence. Each option may be used once, more than once, or not at all.

A   Nothing
B   Aspirin
C   Warfarin
D   Aspirin and warfarin together
E   Heparin
F   Newer anticoagulants, e.g. dabigatran
G CHA_2DS_2VaSc score
H $CHADS_2$ score
I   HAS-BLED score

20-26. Medical management of a breast lump

```
                    ┌─────────────────┐
                    │  Breast lump    │
                    └────────┬────────┘
                             ▼
                    ┌─────────────────┐
                    │  (20) ........   │
                    └────────┬────────┘
          ┌──────────────────┼──────────────────────┐
          ▼                  ▼                       ▼
   ┌────────────┐    ┌─────────────┐        ┌────────────────┐
   │  No lump   │    │  Definite   │        │   Dominant     │
   │            │    │  lump       │        │  asymmetrical  │
   └─────┬──────┘    └──────┬──────┘        │  nodularity    │
         ▼                  ▼               └────────┬───────┘
   ┌────────────┐    ┌─────────────┐                 │
   │ (21) ......│    │ (22) ......  │                 │
   └────────────┘    └─────────────┘      ┌───────────┴──────────┐
                                          ▼                      ▼
                                   ┌────────────┐        ┌────────────────┐
                                   │ <35 y with │        │ ≥35 y or <35 y │
                                   │ no family  │        │ with strong    │
                                   │ history    │        │ family history │
                                   └─────┬──────┘        └───────┬────────┘
                                         ▼                       ▼
                                   ┌────────────┐        ┌────────────────┐
                                   │ (23) ......│        │  (26) ........ │
                                   └─────┬──────┘        └────────────────┘
                              ┌──────────┴─────────┐
                              ▼                    ▼
                       ┌────────────┐       ┌────────────┐
                       │  Persists  │       │  Resolves  │
                       └─────┬──────┘       └─────┬──────┘
                             ▼                    ▼
                       ┌────────────┐       ┌────────────┐
                       │ (24) ......│       │ (25) ......│
                       └────────────┘       └────────────┘
```

For each of the numbered gaps above, select one option from the list below to complete the algorithm, based on current evidence.

A History and examination

B Refer

C Reassure

D Review at 6 weeks

E Biopsy

F Wide local excision

G Tamoxifen

27-33. Symptoms and signs suggestive of chronic heart failure

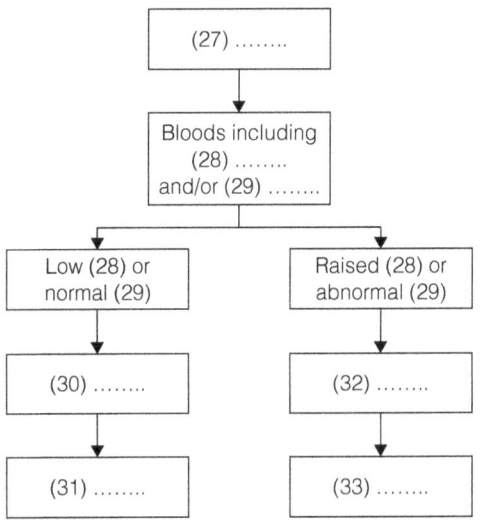

For each of the numbered gaps above, select one option from the list below to complete the algorithm, based on current evidence.

A   History and clinical examination
B   Brain natriuretic peptide
C   Atrial natriuretic peptide
D   Chest X-ray
E   ECG
F   CT scan
G   CHF excluded
H   CHF possible
I   Consider other causes for symptoms
J   Refer to echo to assess cardiac function further

34-39. Pharmacological management of facial hirsutism

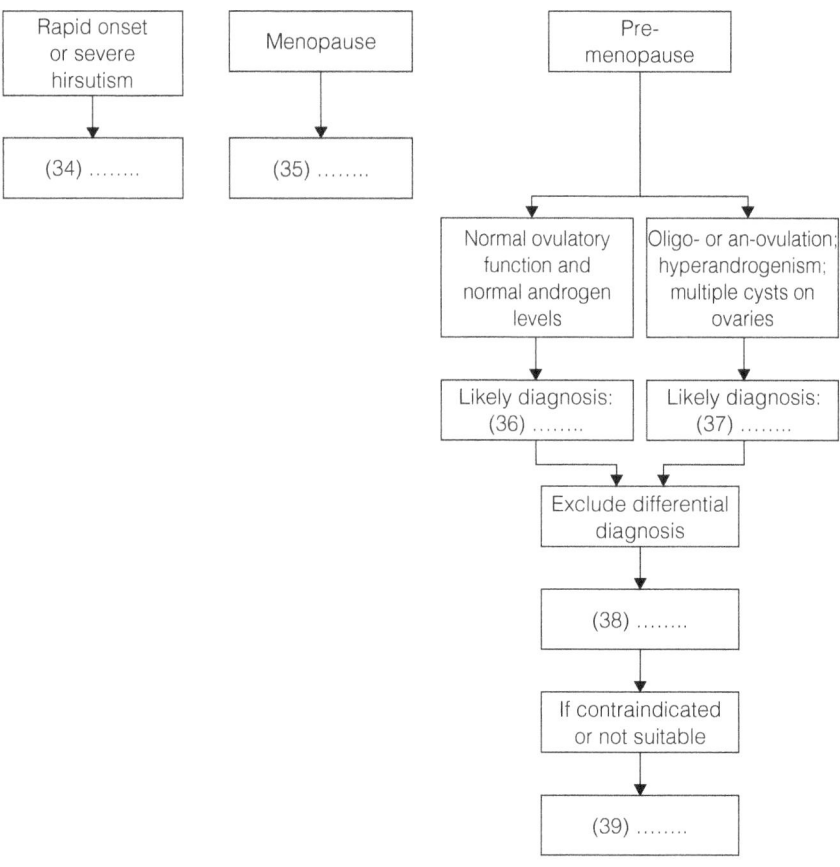

For each of the numbered gaps above, select one option from the list below to complete the algorithm, based on current evidence.

A Cyproterone acetate / ethinyl estradiol
B Refer
C PCOS
D Idiopathic hirsutism
E Eflornithine cream
F Thiazide diuretics

40-52. Choosing drugs for patients newly diagnosed with hypertension

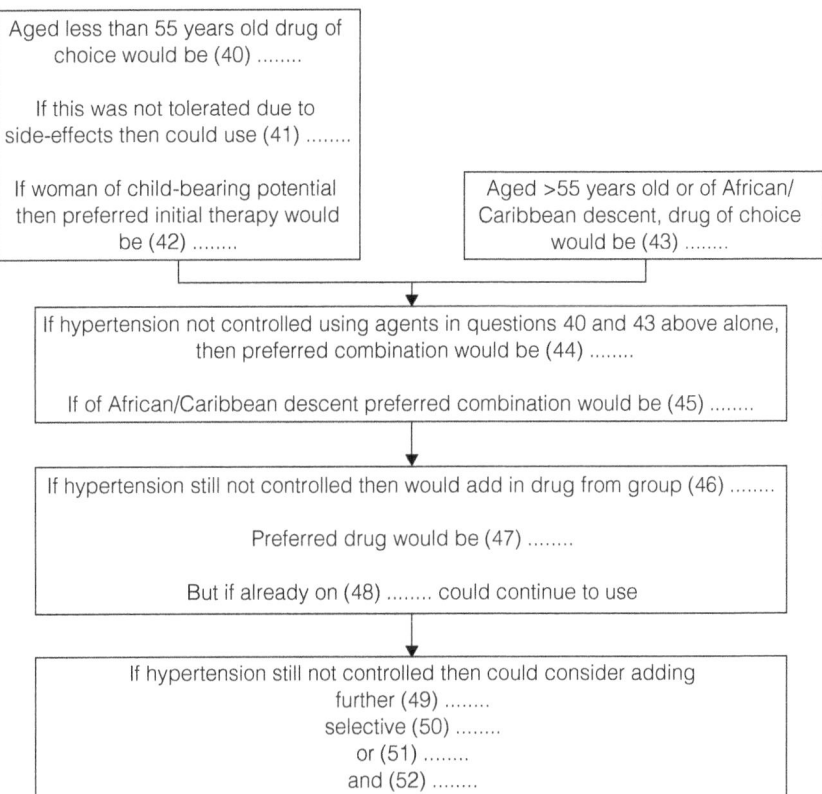

Aged less than 55 years old drug of choice would be (40) ....

If this was not tolerated due to side-effects then could use (41) ....

If woman of child-bearing potential then preferred initial therapy would be (42) ....

Aged >55 years old or of African/Caribbean descent, drug of choice would be (43) ....

If hypertension not controlled using agents in questions 40 and 43 above alone, then preferred combination would be (44) ....

If of African/Caribbean descent preferred combination would be (45) ....

If hypertension still not controlled then would add in drug from group (46) ....

Preferred drug would be (47) ....

But if already on (48) .... could continue to use

If hypertension still not controlled then could consider adding further (49) .... selective (50) .... or (51) .... and (52) ....

For each of the numbered gaps above, select one option from the list below to complete the algorithm, based on current evidence. Each option may be used once, more than once, or not at all. Note: there is more than one possible answer to at least one of the questions.

A Angiotensin II receptor antagonist
B Angiotensin converting enzyme inhibitor
C Beta blocker
D Calcium antagonists
E Angiotensin II receptor antagonist plus calcium antagonist
F Angiotensin converting enzyme inhibitor plus calcium antagonist
G Thiazide diuretic
H Thiazide-like diuretic
I Further diuretic
J Selective alpha blocker
K Indapamide or chlorthalidone
L Bendrofluazide
M Consider seeking expert medical advice

53-60. Management of an unconscious adult

```
┌─────────────────┐
│  Having checked │
│   for hazards   │
└────────┬────────┘
         ▼
┌─────────────────┐
│   (53) ........ │
└────────┬────────┘
         │ Nil
         ▼
┌─────────────────┐
│   (54) ........ │
└────────┬────────┘
         ▼
┌─────────────────┐      ┌──────────┐      ┌──────────────┐
│   (55) ........ │─────▶│ present  │─────▶│  (58) ...... │
└────────┬────────┘      └──────────┘      └──────────────┘
         ▼
┌─────────────────┐
│   (56) ........ │
└────────┬────────┘
         ▼
┌─────────────────┐
│   (57) ........ │
└────────┬────────┘
         ▼
┌─────────────────┐
│   (59) ........ │
└────────┬────────┘
         ▼
┌─────────────────┐
│   (60) ........ │
└─────────────────┘
```

For each of the numbered gaps above, select one option from the list below to complete the algorithm, based on current evidence.

A   Assess for 10 sec
B   Check responsiveness
C   Two effective breaths
D   Open airway by head tilt, chin lift
E   Check breathing
F   Assess for 1 min
G   If breathing, place in recovery position
H   Continue rescue breathing, check circulation every minute
I   Begin chest compressions
J   CPR rate: 5 chest compressions per 1 rescue breath
K   CPR rate: 15 : 2
L   Call 999 for help
M   30 chest compressions
N   CPR rate: 30 : 2

61-64. Coeliac disease care pathway

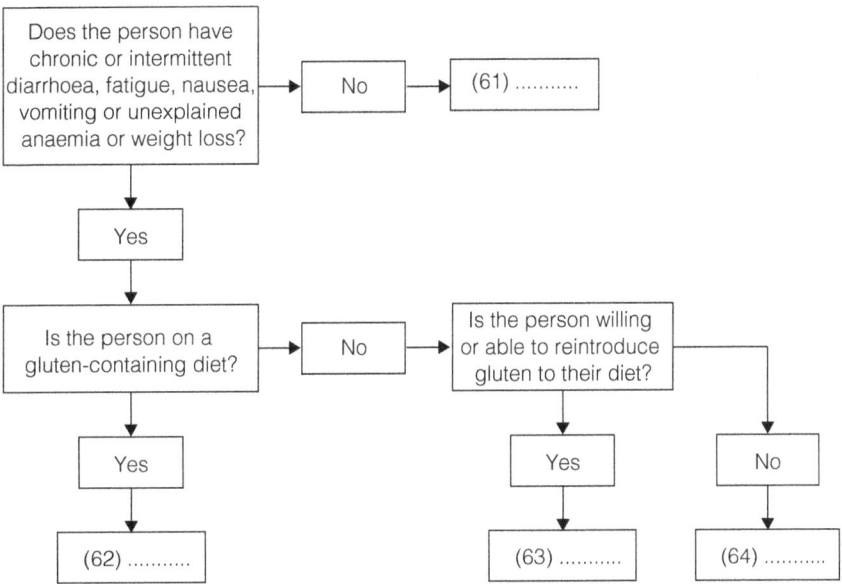

For each of the numbered gaps above, select one option from the list below to complete the algorithm, based on current evidence.

A Refer them to a gastrointestinal specialist and inform them that it may be difficult to make a diagnosis of coeliac disease on biopsy and this may have implications on their ability to access prescribed gluten-free foods

B Offer serological testing

C Person is unlikely to need testing for coeliac disease at this point unless there is a continuing medical problem or symptoms persist

D None of the above

65-71. Management of primary hypothyroidism in non-pregnant adults

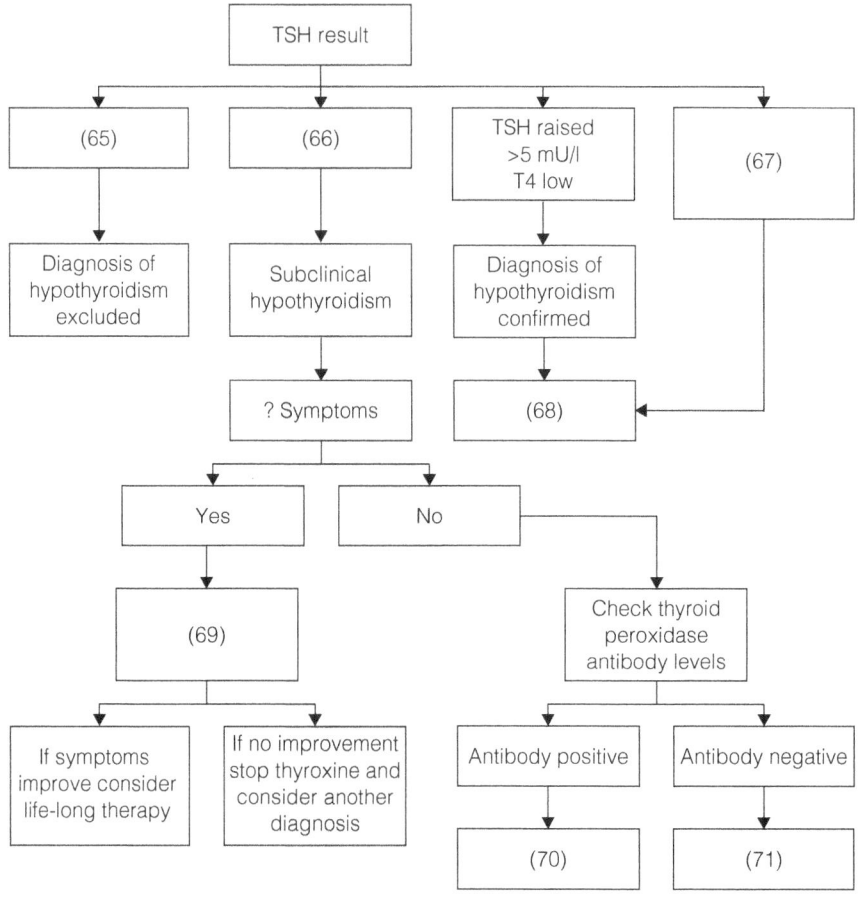

For each of the numbered gaps above, select one option from the list below to complete the algorithm, based on current evidence.

A   Monitor TSH three yearly

B   Offer trial of levothyroxine for 3-6 months and review

C   Monitor TSH annually

D   TSH normal

E   TSH raised >5 mU/l; T4 normal

F   Treat with levothyroxine life-long

G   TSH raised >10 mU/l with or without low free serum thyroxine

72-77. Patients with suspected ovarian cancer

For each of the numbered gaps above, select one option from the list below to complete the algorithm, based on current evidence. Each option may be used once, more than once, or not at all.

A   Refer urgently to secondary care

B   Measure BRCA1

C   Measure BRCA2

D   Measure serum CA125

E   Is aged ≥50 and has had symptoms within the last 12 months that suggest IBS

F   Urgent ultrasound of pelvis

G   Advise woman to return if symptoms become more frequent / persistent

H   Investigate further

Answers to algorithm questions 1-77

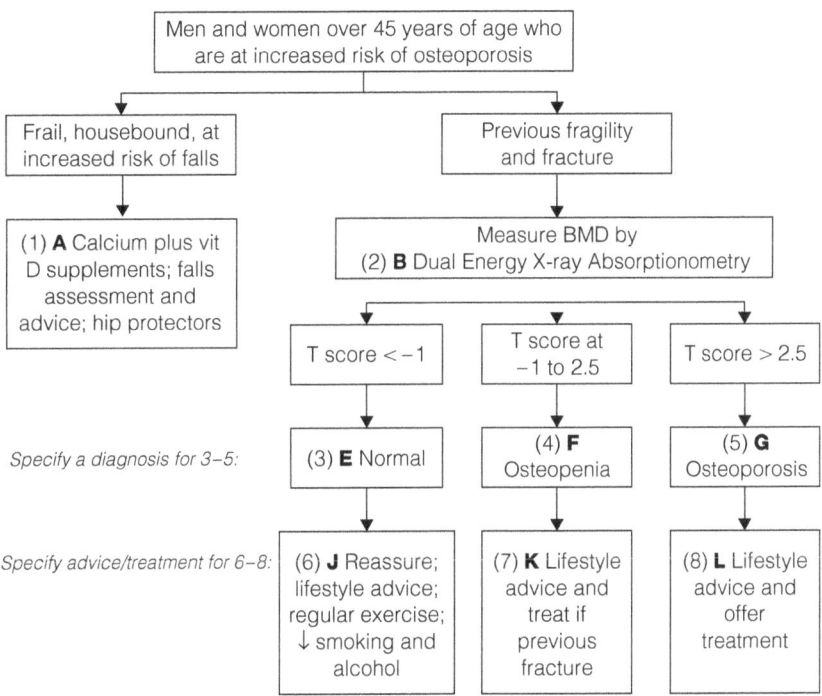

Men and women over 45 years of age who are at increased risk of osteoporosis

Frail, housebound, at increased risk of falls

Previous fragility and fracture

(1) **A** Calcium plus vit D supplements; falls assessment and advice; hip protectors

Measure BMD by
(2) **B** Dual Energy X-ray Absorptionometry

T score < −1

T score at −1 to 2.5

T score > 2.5

Specify a diagnosis for 3–5:

(3) **E** Normal

(4) **F** Osteopenia

(5) **G** Osteoporosis

Specify advice/treatment for 6–8:

(6) **J** Reassure; lifestyle advice; regular exercise; ↓ smoking and alcohol

(7) **K** Lifestyle advice and treat if previous fracture

(8) **L** Lifestyle advice and offer treatment

1. **Answer is A.**
2. **Answer is B.**
3. **Answer is E.**
4. **Answer is F.**
5. **Answer is G.**
6. **Answer is J.**
7. **Answer is K.**
8. **Answer is L.**

Answers to questions 1–8 are all drawn from Royal College of Physicians and Bone and Tooth Society of Great Britain (July 2005): *Osteoporosis – clinical guidelines for prevention and treatment.*

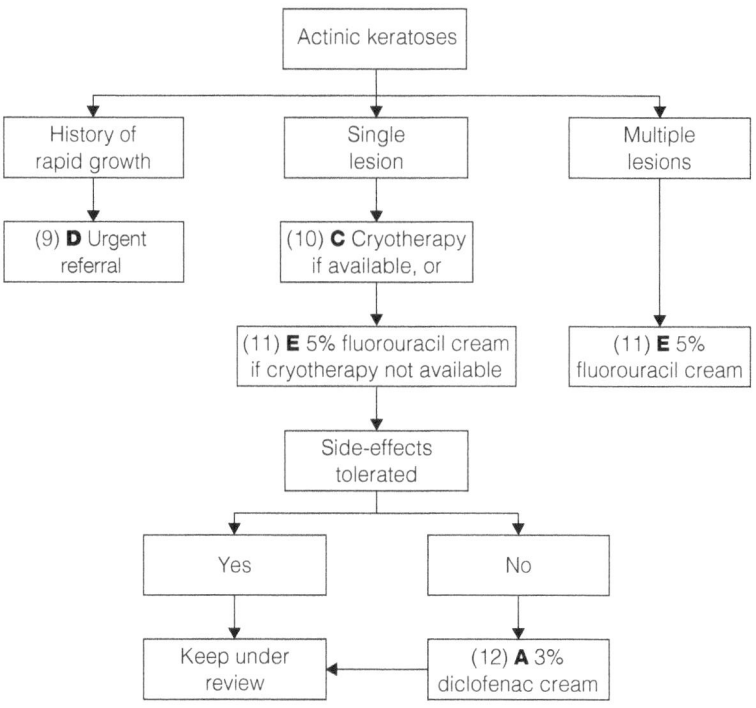

9. **Answer is D.**
10. **Answer is C.**
11. **Answer is E.**
12. **Answer is A.**

Answers to questions 9–12 drawn from Working Party Guidelines (2004): *The primary and shared care management of actinic keratoses.*

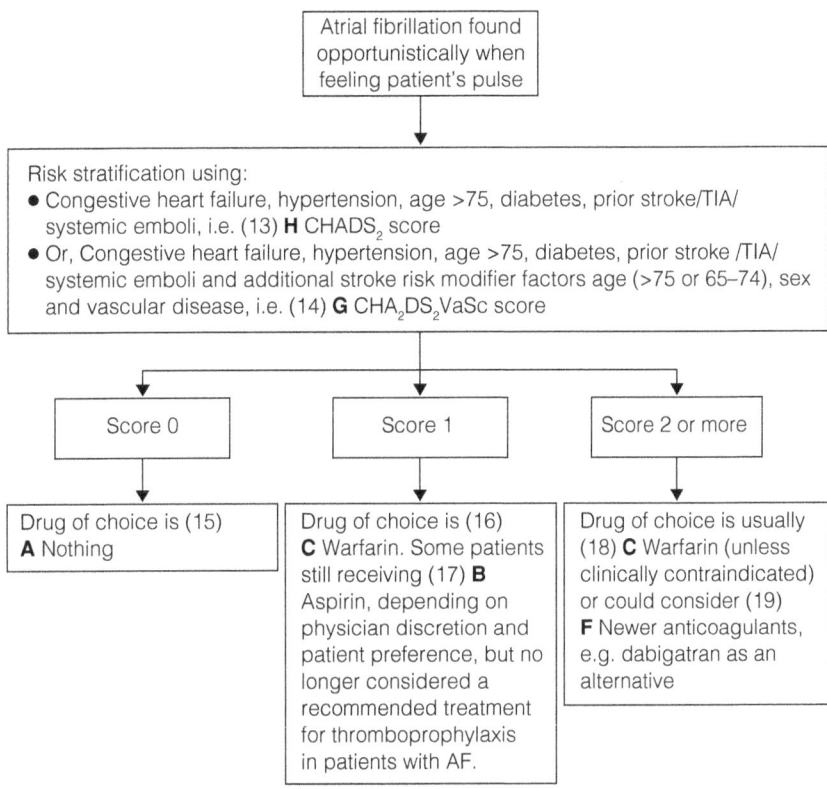

13. **Answer is H.**
14. **Answer is G.**
15. **Answer is A.**
16. **Answer is C.**
17. **Answer is B.**
18. **Answer is C.**
19. **Answer is F.**

Answers to questions 13–19 are drawn from *NICE CG36, The management of atrial fibrillation* (www.nice.org.uk/CG36). The original guidance was published in 2006. Since then further changes have been introduced; from April 2012 QOF requires all with AF to be stratified annually for stroke risk using the CHADS$_2$ tool and using this to decide regarding antithrombotic therapy based on age; the other change has been the approval of dabigatran and rivaroxaban for thromboprophylaxis in AF.

SIGN 129: *Antithrombotics: indications and management, Quick Reference Guide* (updated June 2013) is more up to date.

Aspirin is currently still recognised by QOF and NICE guidelines but is no longer a recommended treatment for thromboprophylaxis in patients with AF (*BMJ* 2013; **346:** f3719).

(The HAS-BLED scoring system is used to identify patients at increased risk of haemorrhage.)

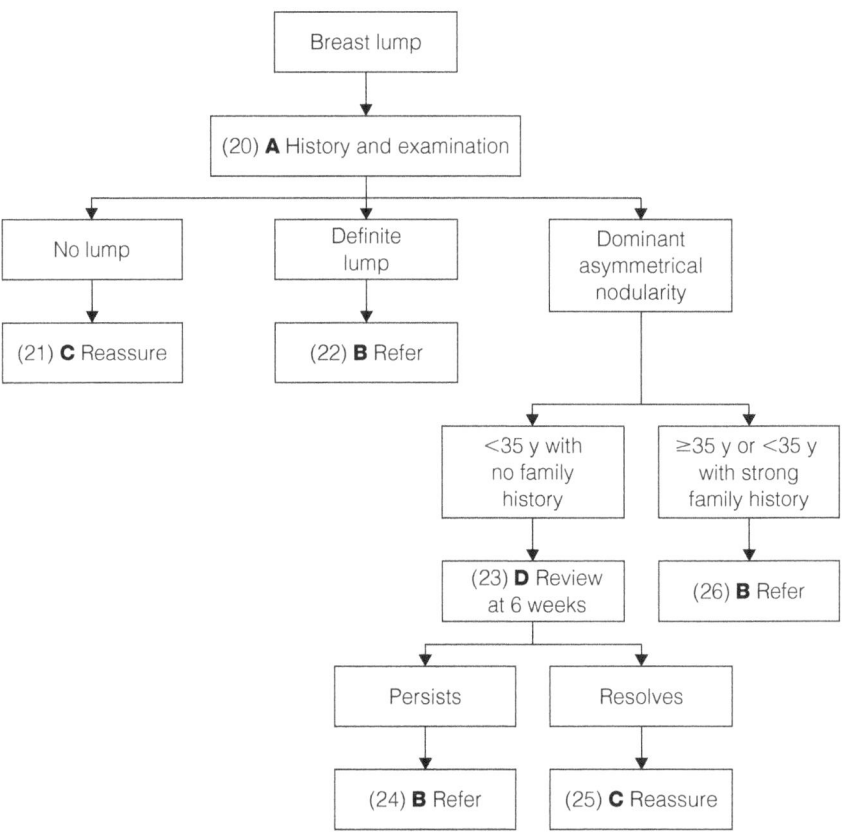

20. Answer is A.
21. Answer is C.
22. Answer is B.
23. Answer is D.
24. Answer is B.
25. Answer is C.
26. Answer is B.

Answers to questions 20–26 are all drawn from:
- NHS Cancer Screening Programmes and Cancer Research UK (2003) *Guidelines for referral of patients with breast problems*
- *NICE Clinical Guidelines* (August 2002) *Improving outcomes in breast cancer*

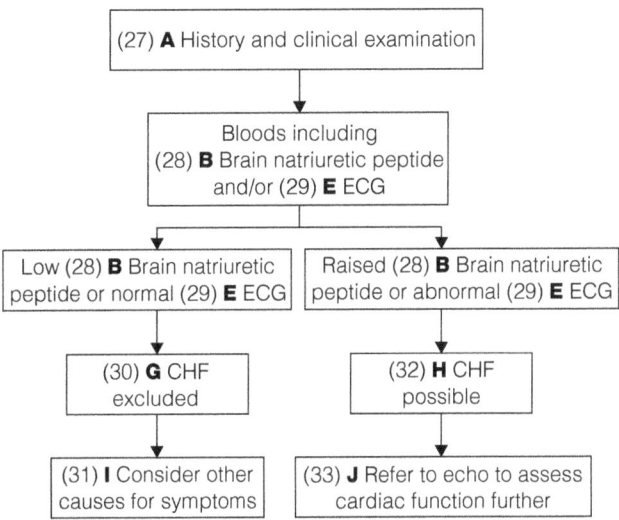

27. Answer is A.

28. Answer is B.

29. Answer is E.

30. Answer is G.

31. Answer is I.

32. Answer is H.

33. Answer is J.

Answers to questions 27–33 are all drawn from:

- *NICE Clinical Guidelines* (July 2003)
- *European Heart Journal* 2005; **26**: 1115–40 – *Guidelines for the diagnosis and treatment of chronic heart failure* – European Society of Cardiology

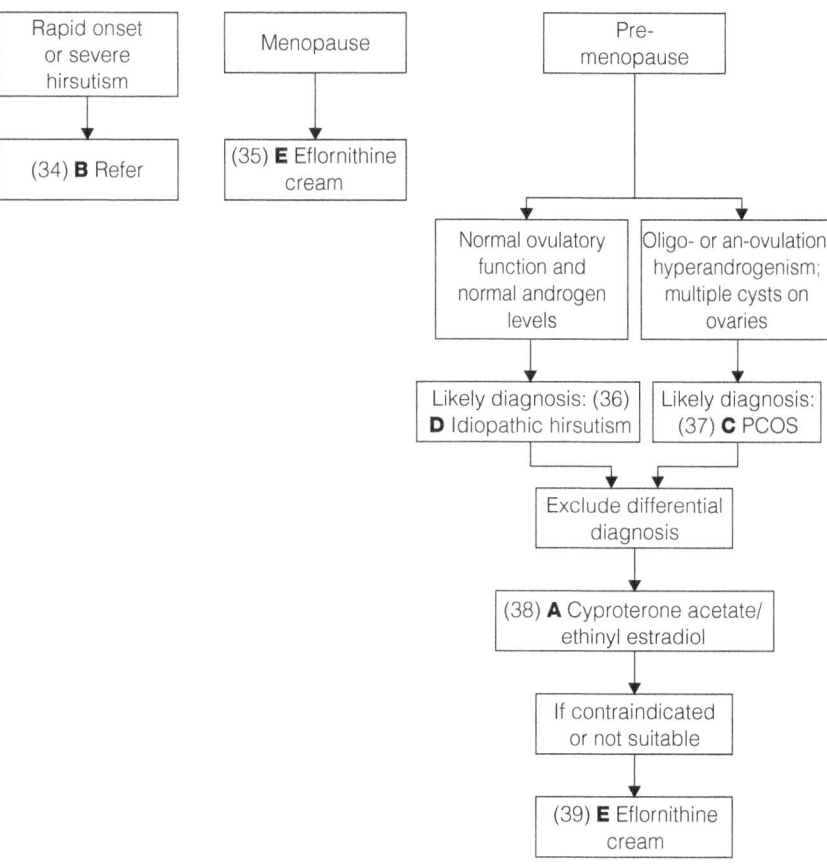

34. Answer is B.

35. Answer is E.

36. Answer is D.

37. Answer is C.

38. Answer is A.

39. Answer is E.

All answers drawn from www.eguidelines.co.uk/eguidelinesmain/guidelines/summaries/skin/wp_facial_hirsutism.php [accessed 1 July 2013] *Medical management of facial hirsutism: working party guidelines.*

Aged less than 55 years old drug of choice would be (40) **B** Angiotensin converting enzyme inhibitor

If this was not tolerated due to side-effects then could use (41) **A** Angiotensin II receptor antagonist

If woman of child-bearing potential then preferred initial therapy would be (42) **C** Beta blocker

Aged >55 years old or of African/Caribbean descent, drug of choice would be (43) **D** Calcium antagonists

↓

If hypertension not controlled using agents in questions 40 and 43 above alone, then preferred combination would be (44) **F** Angiotensin converting enzyme inhibitor plus calcium antagonist

If of African/Caribbean descent preferred combination would be (45) **E** Angiotensin II receptor antagonist plus calcium antagonist

↓

If hypertension still not controlled then would add in drug from group (46) **H** Thiazide-like diuretic

Preferred drug would be (47) **K** Indapamide or chlorthalidone

But if already on (48) **L** Bendrofluazide or **G** Thiazide diuretic could continue to use

↓

If hypertension still not controlled then could consider adding further (49) **L** Bendrofluazide selective (50) **J** Selective alpha blocker or (51) **C** Beta blocker and (52) **M** Consider seeking expert medical advice

40. Answer is B.
41. Answer is A.
42. Answer is C.
43. Answer is D.
44. Answer is F.
45. Answer is E.
46. Answer is H.
47. Answer is K.
48. Answer is L or G.
49. Answer is L.
50. Answer is J.
51. Answer is C.
52. Answer is M.

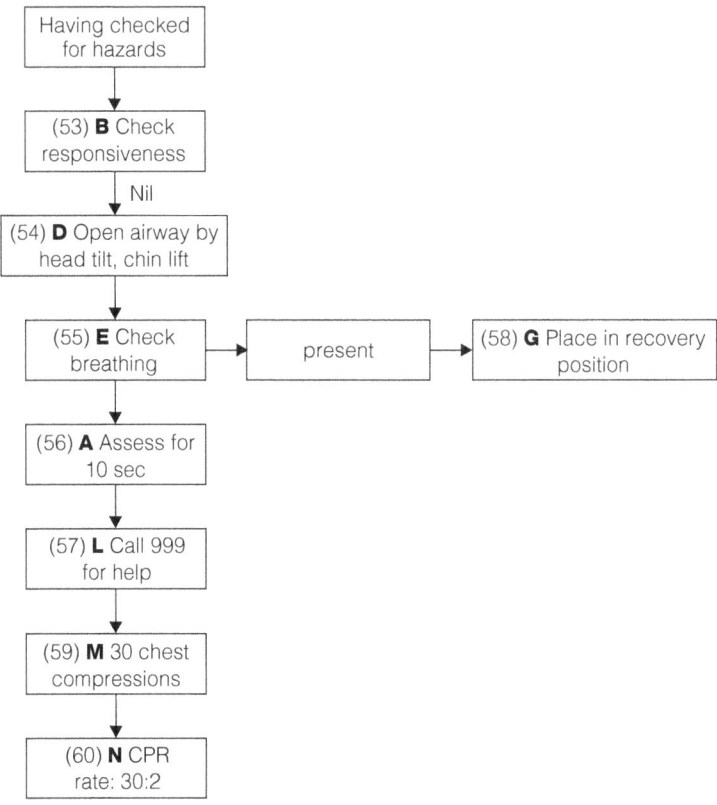

53. Answer is B.
54. Answer is D.
55. Answer is E.
56. Answer is A.
57. Answer is L.
58. Answer is G.
59. Answer is M.
60. Answer is N.

Answers to questions 53–60 are all drawn from *Resuscitation Council (UK) Guidelines* (2005).

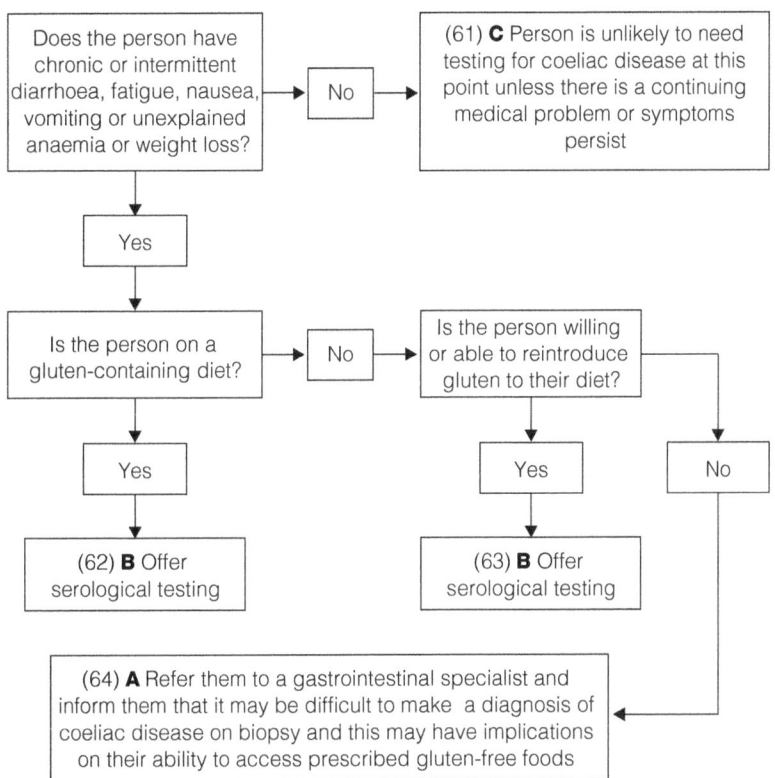

61. Answer is C.
62. Answer is B.
63. Answer is B.
64. Answer is A.

    Answers to questions 61–64 are all drawn from *NICE Guideline CG86: Coeliac disease: recognition and assessment of coeliac disease* (May 2009).

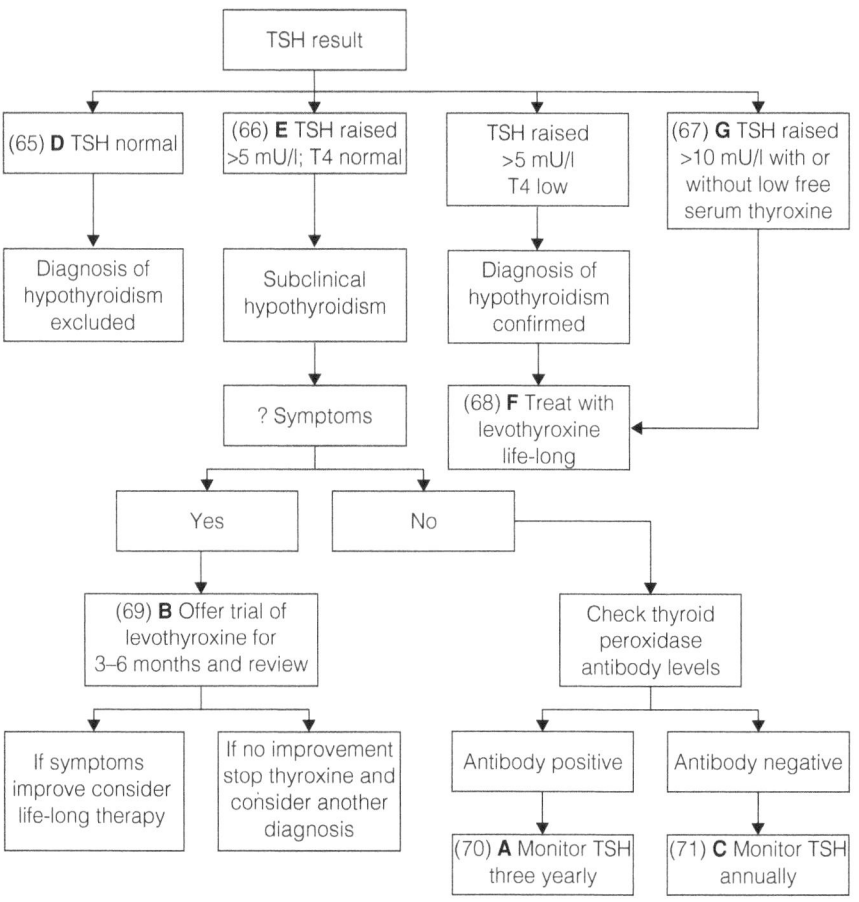

65. **Answer is D.**
66. **Answer is E.**
67. **Answer is G.**
68. **Answer is F.**
69. **Answer is B.**
70. **Answer is A.**
71. **Answer is C.**

The evidence base for when to treat subclinical hypothyroidism is not well developed and is based on expert consensus; the rationale for treatment is that 2–4% progress to overt hypothyroidism annually and that patients may have symptoms of underactive thyroid which impair quality of life, even in the presence of normal T3/4.

The exception to the above is in pregnancy or in those trying to conceive, when subclinical hypothyroidism should always be treated and referred for shared obstetric care.

Answers to questions 65–71 are based on best practice as outlined in *BMJ*, 2008, **337:** A801.

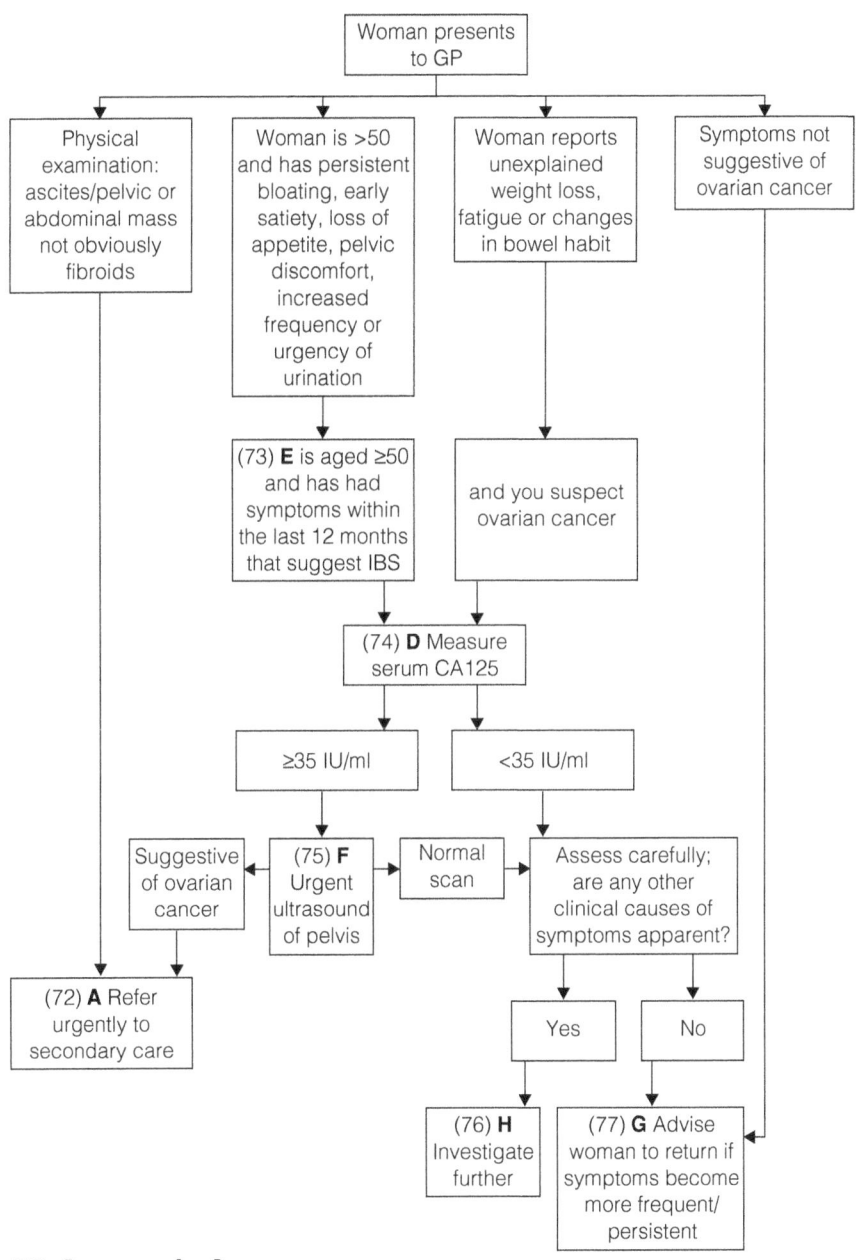

72. **Answer is A.**
73. **Answer is E.**
74. **Answer is D.**
75. **Answer is F.**
76. **Answer is H.**
77. **Answer is G.**

Answers to questions 72–77 are all drawn from *NICE Clinical Guideline 122, April 2011, The recognition and initial management of ovarian cancer.*

Picture questions 1-47

for answers see pages 165–172

1. Skin rash

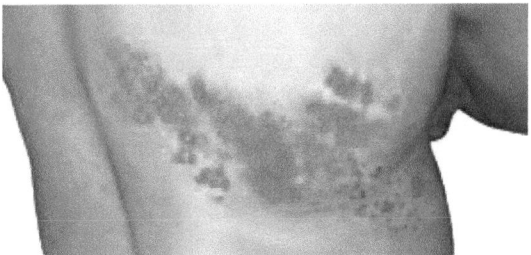

With regard to this rash choose one correct answer from the list below:

A Typically painless

B Typically seen in fit healthy young men

C It is due to herpes simplex virus type 2

D Topical lidocaine is not recommended as a first-line agent in the treatment of post rash complications

E Reduced in terms of duration and severity of pain if systemic antiviral treatment is started within 4 to 8 days after presentation

2. Skin rash

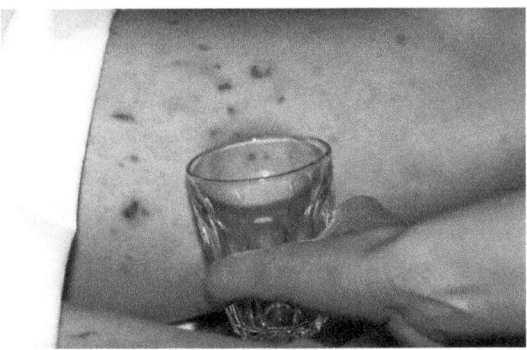

Which one of the following statements is true?

A Early signs of this disease in children include leg pains, cold hands/feet and a mottled skin colour

B Oral penicillin should be given before hospital admission by the GP

C This non-blanching haemorrhagic purple rash is due to chicken pox virus

D In children, the classic symptoms of this disease (i.e. rash, headache and impaired consciousness) always appear within the first 2 hours of the illness

E IV penicillin should be given before hospital admission by the GP

F The GP should then personally arrange contact tracing and prophylaxis for the family and kissing contacts.

3-6. Systematic review and meta analysis

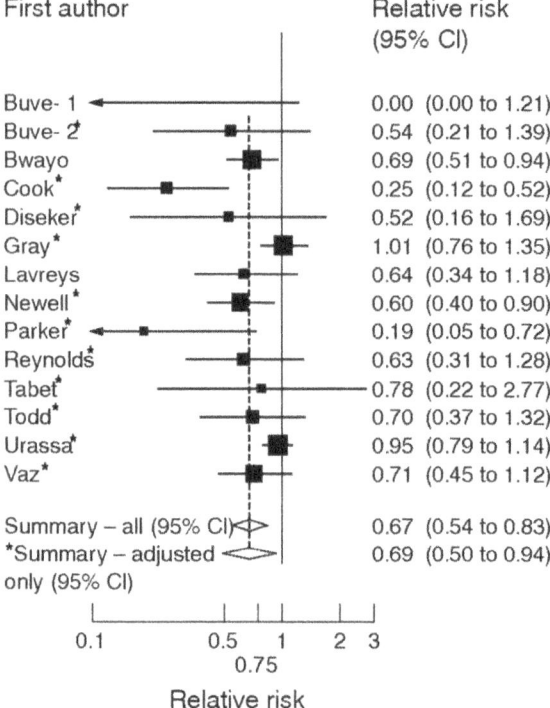

A   Horizontal line (there are 14 shown)
B   Square in middle of each horizontal line
C   Width of each horizontal line
D   Solid vertical line down middle
E   Diamond below all horizontal lines (there are two here)

Considering the systematic review and meta analysis data shown above, match the definitions to the description given; each definition may be used only once, and not all of them are used.

3.   This sign represents pooled data from all trials shown.

4.   This represents the 95% confidence interval of this estimate.

5.   This is the line of no effect and is associated with a relative risk of 1.0.

6.   This corresponds to each trial and shows the relative risk of the condition as a result of the intervention.

7. Device failure

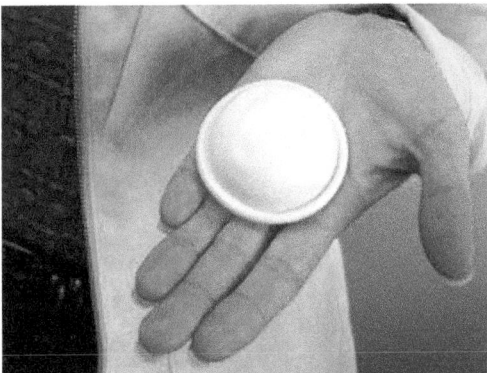

Which one of the following does not affect the failure rate of this device?

A   Petroleum jelly
B   Vaseline
C   Baby oil
D   Clotrimazole cream 1%
E   KY jelly

8. Ophthalmology

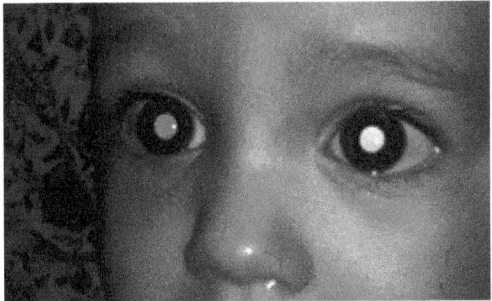

The mother of a two year old child brings her to see you; she has brought with her a number of recent photos, including the one shown above; the child is well and asymptomatic; on examination with an ophthalmoscope you are unable to elicit a red reflex in the left eye.

Which one of the following is true?

A   The child should be reviewed by yourself in two weeks
B   It most likely be a problem with the camera which should be replaced and the child re-photographed
C   The child should be referred routinely
D   The condition could be lethal
E   The condition is never hereditary

9. Ophthalmology

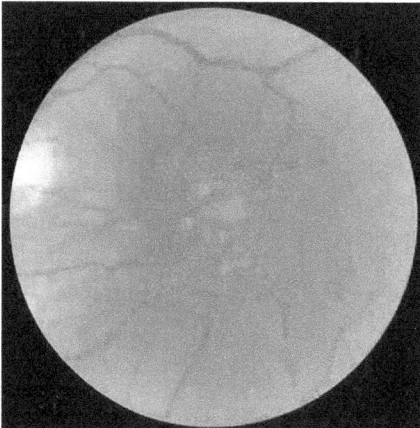

Which one of the following statements concerning this photograph is correct?

A This is a photo showing panretinal photocoagulation scars in a patient with diabetic retinopathy

B The white spots are small haemorrhages

C This picture is typical of wet age-related macular degeneration

D This picture is typical of dry age-related macular degeneration

E The deposits are covering the optic nerve

10. ECG

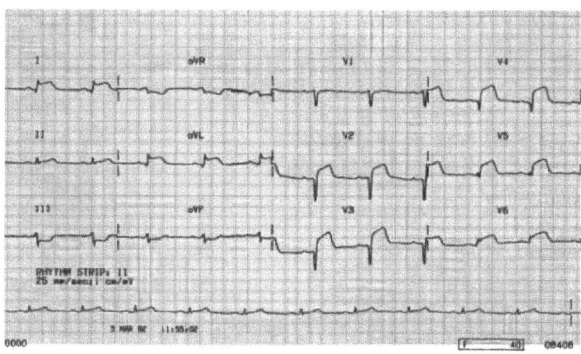

A 40 year old man collapses with chest pain; his ECG shown above displays which one of the following?

A Acute anterior myocardial infarction

B Acute postero–inferior myocardial infarction

C Old anterior myocardial infarction

D Pulmonary embolism

E Normal ECG

11. Facial weakness

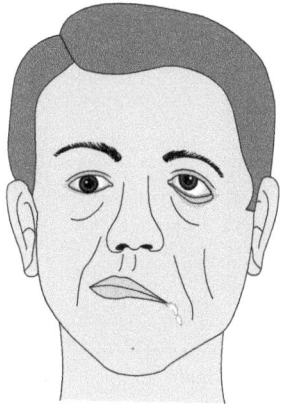

A fit and healthy, non-smoking 26 year old man attends with sudden onset of weakness affecting the left side of his face; he has a smooth forehead and is dribbling from the left side of his mouth; he is unable to close his left eye. His grandfather recently had a stroke at the age of 66 years. He looks as shown in the diagram above.

Further examination reveals a crop of vesicles affecting the external auditory meatus of the left ear and he has developed a sensitivity to loud sounds.

Which one of the following is true?
A This man has had a stroke and needs to be referred to a stroke unit
B This man has herpes zoster oticus
C He has an upper motor lesion affecting the facial cranial nerve
D He has a lower motor lesion affecting the tenth
E Taste disturbance affecting the ipsilateral 2/3 of the tongue is uncommon

12. Oral mucosal discolouration

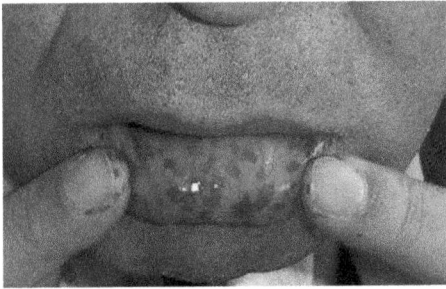

What does this photograph illustrate?
A Peutz–Jeghers syndrome
B Acanthosis nigricans
C Hereditary haemorrhagic telangiectasia
D Addison's disease

13. Skin rash

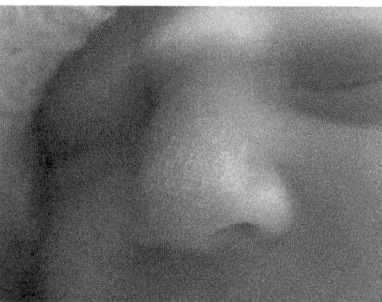

A first time mum attends with her two week old child worried about a rash (as shown in the photograph above) on her baby's nose.

Which one of the following options is the correct management of these small white spots?

A Mild topical steroid for two weeks
B 1% clotrimazole
C Pierce with orange stick
D Nothing
E Curettage

14. Musculoskeletal

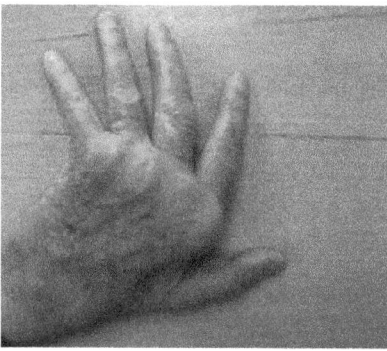

Considering the photograph above, which one of the following statements is true?

A The patient is unlikely to have systemic involvement
B Early diagnosis and treatment are crucial to avoid irreversible damage to the joints
C Anti-cyclic citrullinated peptide antibodies are not highly specific for this disease
D If a patient is treated with biological agents, they need to be informed that treatment will be lifelong and they are unlikely to be taken off such medication once it has been initiated
E The patient is more likely to be male than female

15. Dermatology

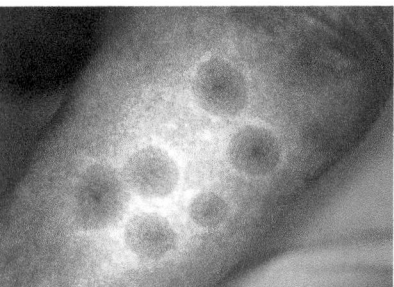

An 18 year old man who was prescribed a course of antibiotics for a sore throat last week, saw one of your colleagues yesterday when he developed these lesions on his forearms; they appeared suddenly, starting as small flat red spots that enlarged over the next day or so, the central area cleared and now looks pale purple; they are minimally itchy and not painful. However, the rash has spread proximally and although he is well, he is concerned that he may have chicken pox.

Which one of the following best describes this picture?

A   Erythema nodosum
B   Erythema multiforme
C   Vitiligo
D   Erythema ab igne
E   Erythrasma

16. Dermatology

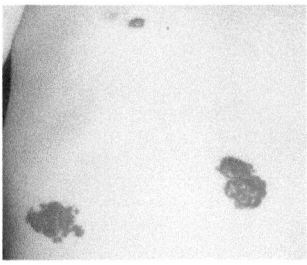

An anxious mother brings her 4 week old daughter; she has developed these small lesions on her abdomen; the mother is certain they were not there when the baby was born and is worried they are getting bigger. Physical examination of the baby is otherwise normal.

Which one of the following should you advise in terms of treatment?

A   Topical fusidic acid
B   Salicylic acid
C   Clotrimazole
D   Topical silver nitrate
E   Nothing

17. ENT

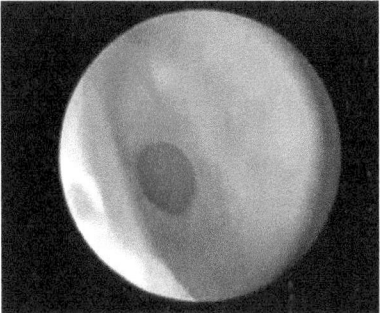

Which one of the following best describes the photograph above?

A   Perforated ear drum
B   Normal tympanic membrane
C   Cholesteatoma
D   Grommet *in situ*
E   Wax

18. Ophthalmology

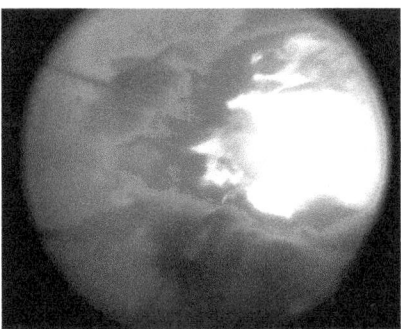

A 61 year old lady, who has been a poorly controlled diabetic for 26 years, comes to you worried; she awoke that morning with a sudden onset of misty vision in her right eye: she describes waking up and her vision being like looking through a car windscreen on a rainy day; there was no pain; on examination she is able to see hand movements only with the right eye and VA in the left is 6/9. On ophthalmoscopy, you see the image as shown; the left fundus reveals proliferative retinopathy. BP is 160/90.

Which one of the following best describes what has happened?

A   Vitreous haemorrhage
B   Acute cataract
C   Acute glaucoma
D   Central retinal artery thrombosis
E   Hysterical blindness

19. Toe nails

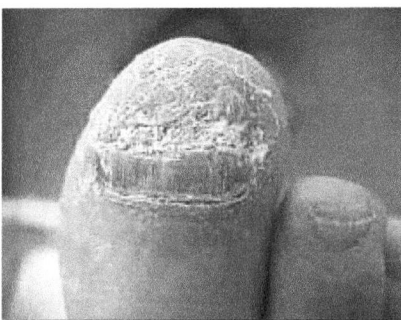

Which one of the following is the best systemic treatment for this condition?

A Terbinafine
B Flucloxacillin
C Fluconazole
D Tea tree oil
E Griseofulvin
F Itraconazole

20. Dermatology

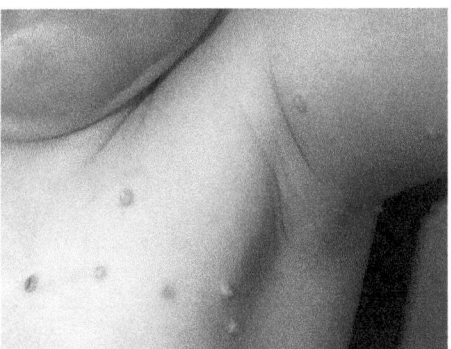

A mother brings her otherwise well 3 year old to see you; she has developed these spots on her chest and, although they do not bother the child, the mother is worried because initially there were only three but they have increased in number. The school nursery has asked that the child be excluded and have told the mother that the little girl has a highly contagious virus; both mother and daughter swim regularly at the local pool.

Which one of the following best describes the condition?

A Seborrhoeic warts
B Molluscum contagiosum
C Chicken pox
D Smallpox

21. Rheumatology

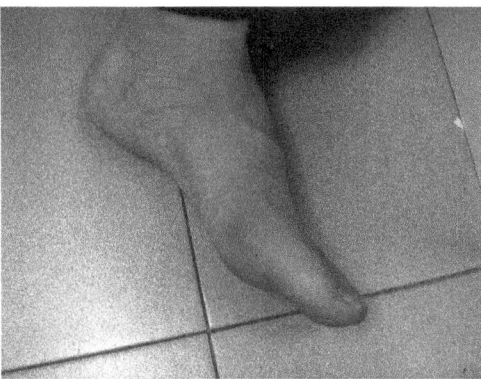

A 58 year old man has requested a house call because of sudden onset intense pain affecting the big toe; he describes it as an excruciating, gnawing sensation and is unable to tolerate even the bed covers on it; he is otherwise fit and well apart from 'a touch of blood pressure' for which he takes bendroflumethiazide 2.5 mg o.d. The clinical picture is as shown in the photograph above.

Which one of the following statements is correct?

A   In the acute phase, where there are no contraindications, fast-acting i.m. NSAIDs are the drugs of choice

B   Colchicine is effective and works as quickly as NSAIDs

C   Allopurinol may be commenced during the acute attack

D   In overweight patients, dieting should be encouraged; a high protein, low carbohydrate diet (e.g. Atkins) is ideal

E   Overall protein intake should be restricted

22. ENT

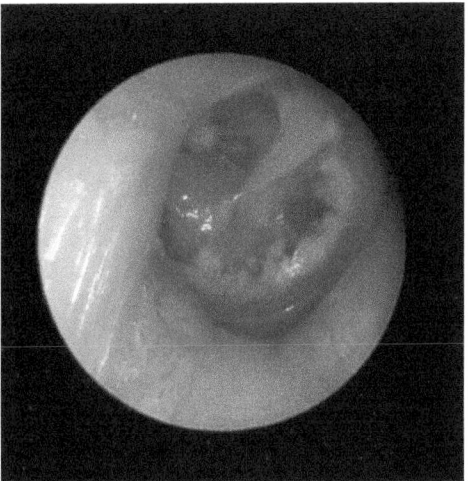

An 18 year old boy attends complaining of deafness, affecting the right ear; this has been getting worse over the past few months; he gives a long history of recurrent otitis media affecting both ears, worse on the right, for which he had grommets on two occasions as a child; there is no tinnitus, vertigo, nystagmus or systemic upset. Examination of the left drum is normal, the right drum is as shown on the photograph above.

Weber's test localises to the right ear and Rinne's test is louder behind the right ear than in front, and louder in front of the left ear than behind.

Which one of the following is true?
A He is likely to have tympanosclerosis
B He should have the deposits on the typanic membrane scraped away with a sharp implement
C He has right sensorineural deafness
D He has left conductive hearing loss

23. ECG

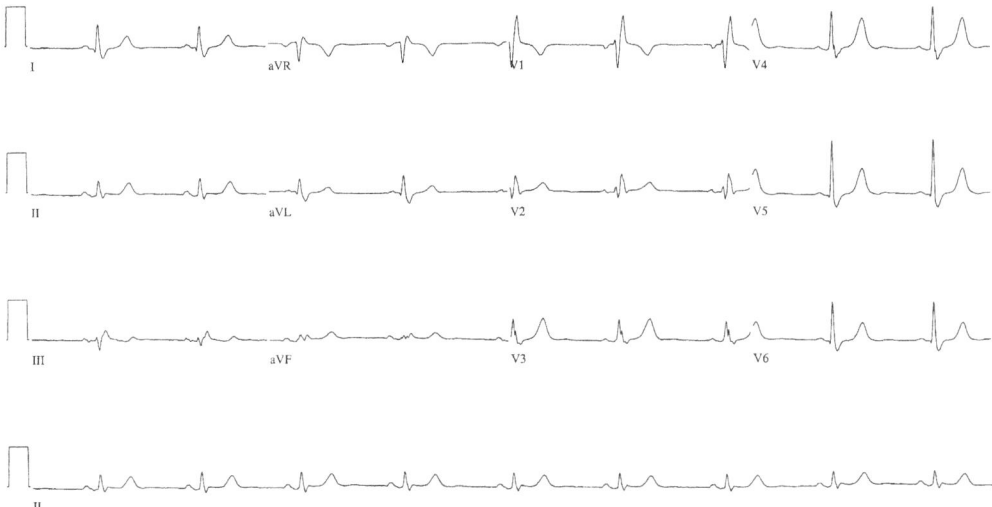

Which one of the following is false in this ECG of a 22 year old male undertaken during a routine medical?

A   The ECG shows left bundle branch block

B   The abnormality shown could be a normal variant in some people

C   The patient is in sinus rhythm

D   The patient needs routine referral to cardiac outpatients for a pacemaker

24-29: Dermatology

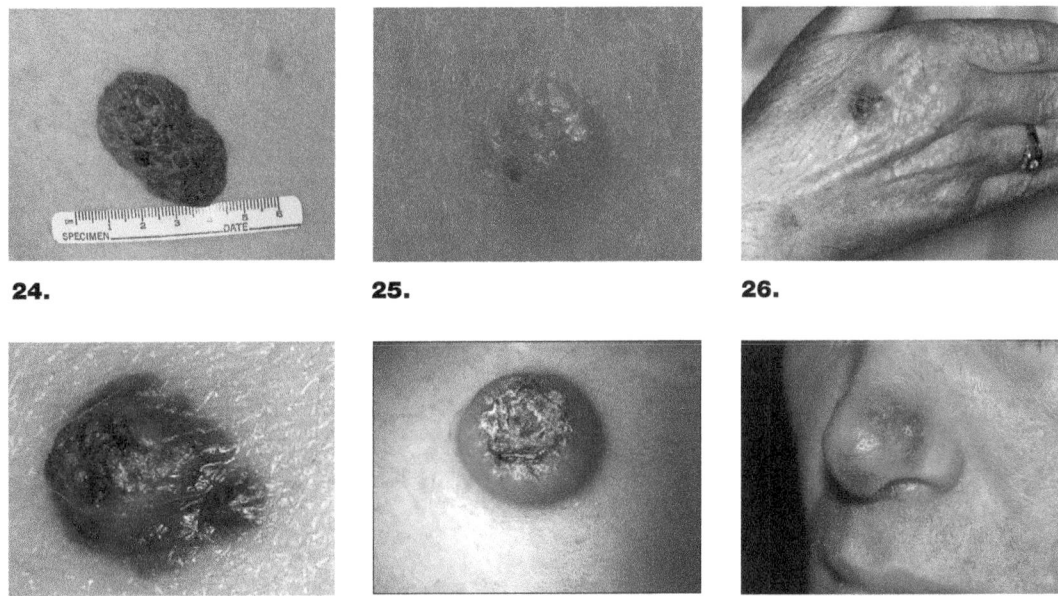

24.

25.

26.

27.

28.

29.

Match the skin lesions below to the correct picture:

A   Basal cell carcinoma
B   Seborrhoeic keratoses
C   Malignant melanoma
D   Keratoacanthoma
E   Squamous cell carcinoma
F   Kaposi's sarcoma

30. Paediatric dermatology

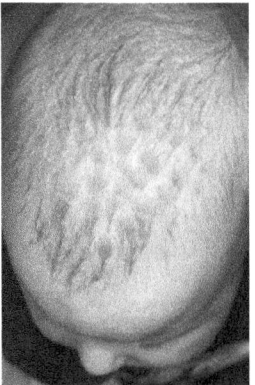

You see an anxious mother for a routine post-natal check; she is becoming increasingly alarmed at the appearance of her son's scalp and would like your advice.

What is the most appropriate management?
A   Take scrapings and send to laboratory
B   Olive oil and baby shampoo
C   Fucithalmic ointment qds
D   Canesten cream bd
E   Refer to dermatology

31. Oral lesions

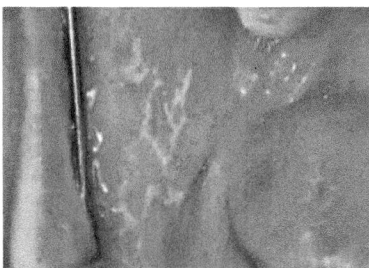

A 50 year old man has been referred to you by his dentist with this oral lesion. He takes allopurinol for gout and is otherwise fit and well.

What is the lesion?
A   Oral thrush
B   Lichen planus
C   Trauma from dentures
D   Koplik's spots
E   Aphthous ulcers

32. Swollen arm

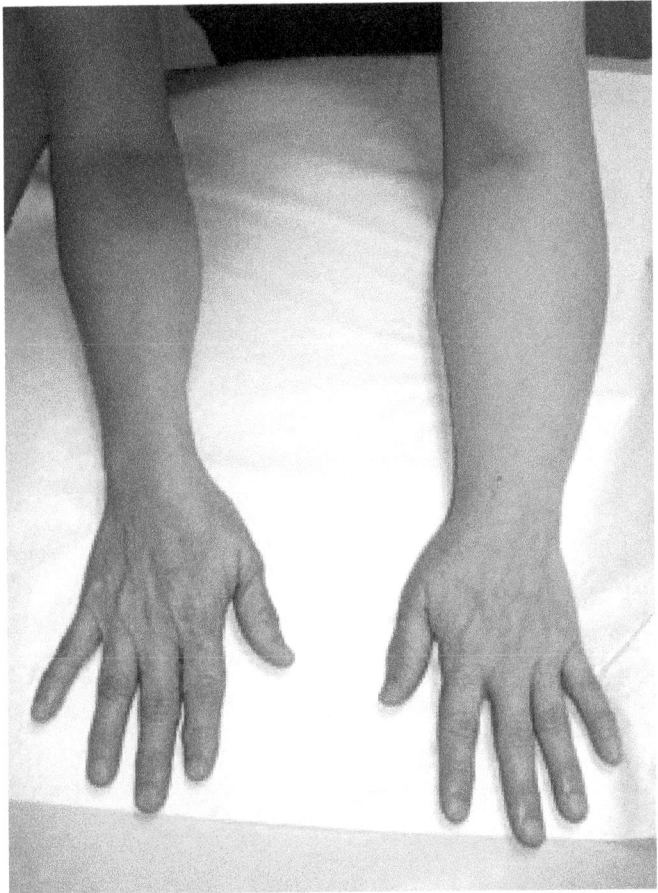

A 66 year old lady attends for hypertension review but is reluctant to let you take the reading from her left arm; she had a mastectomy and axillary clearance for breast cancer three years previously.

You note her left arm is much bigger than her right but the swelling is not tender and the skin does not feel inflamed; she is systemically well.

Which one of the following is the cause of her symptoms?

A DVT
B Cellulitis
C Secondary spread of the malignancy
D Lymphoedema

33-36. Audiograms

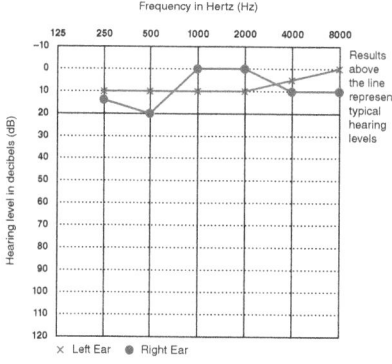

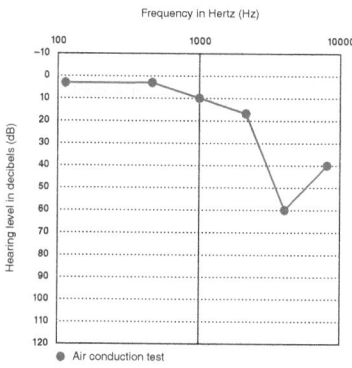

33. A 26 year old housewife

34. A 46 year old factory worker working in a noisy environment since age 16

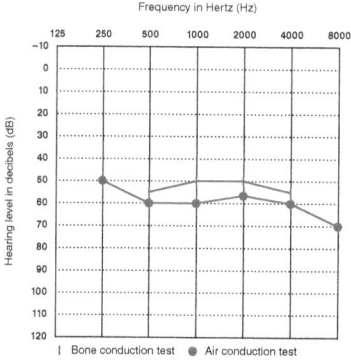

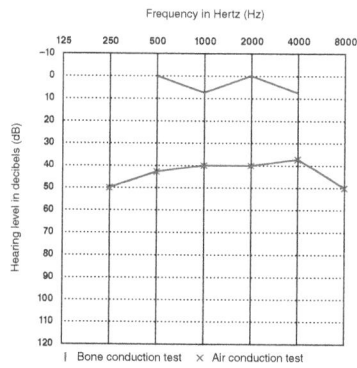

35. An elderly gentleman complaining of deafness in the right ear; known to have Ménière's disease

36. A 6 year old boy with repeated ear infections; these are the results from his left ear

Match the audiogram to the correct label:

A Normal

B Hearing loss after noise damage

C Sensorineural hearing loss

D Conductive hearing loss

37-41. Hearing tests

Look at the series of pictures below of hearing tests being carried out using a 512 Hz tuning fork on an 86 year old gentleman whose wife thinks he may be deaf.

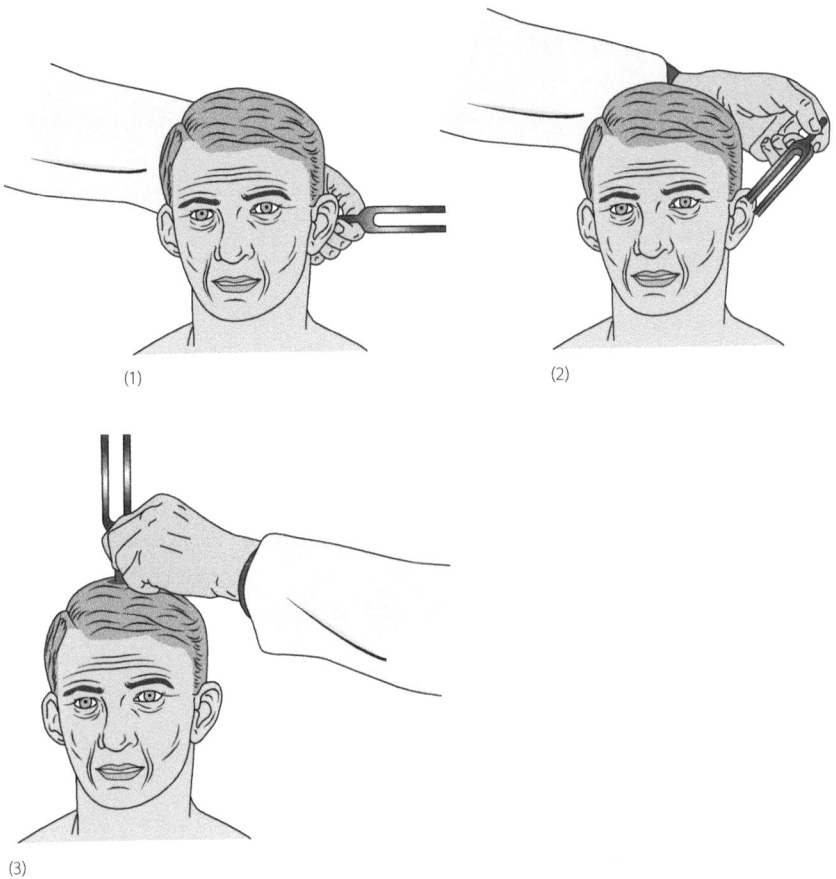

(1)

(2)

(3)

A   Rinne's test
B   Weber's test
C   Conductive deafness of the right ear
D   Conductive deafness of the left ear
E   Normal result
F   Right-sided sensorineural hearing loss
G   Left-sided sensorineural hearing loss

37. *What is the name of the test being carried out in pictures 1 and 2?*

38. *What is the name of the test being carried out in picture 3?*

39. The gentleman reports that he can hear the vibrations of the tuning fork louder in behind his right ear when the fork is placed on the mastoid process than in front at the external auditory meatus and when the fork is placed on his forehead he can hear the vibrations louder on the right side too.

What could be causing this?

40. The gentleman reports he can hear the vibrations louder in front of his right ear than behind and when the fork is held on the forehead the vibrations are equal on both sides.

What can you tell him?

41. If the note is audible at the external meatus when doing the first test, but localises to the left when doing the second test, *what could this be due to?*

42. Child development

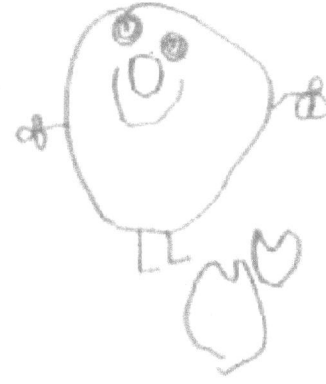

Maisey comes to see you for a repeat prescription of her emollients for eczema; she has drawn a picture for you, shown above.

How old is Maisey likely to be?
A Two years old
B Four years old
C Six years old
D Eight years old

43. ENT

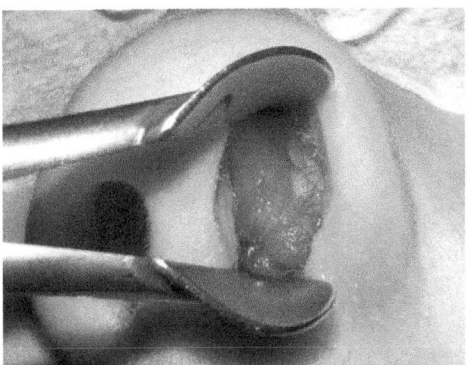

A 40 year old man has a long history of runny nose, especially worse in the spring, for which he has found steroid nasal sprays helpful. He is now presenting with a loss of smell and sensation of blockage but despite using his spray regularly, symptoms persist; he is otherwise well and a non-smoker.

You examine him and find the above bilaterally.

What is this?
A   Nasal polyp
B   Inferior turbinate
C   Foreign body
D   Perforated septum
E   Tumour

44. Oral lesion

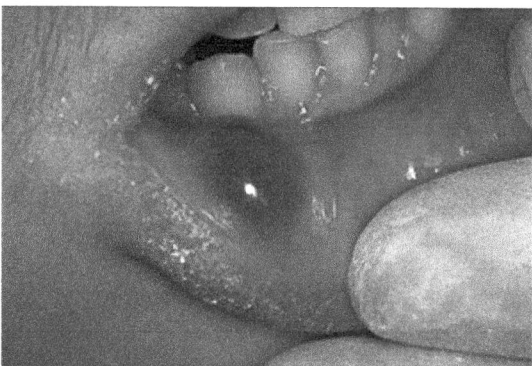

A 43 year old GP colleague of yours presents with the above lesion inside his mouth; he recalls biting the inside of his lip when he was rushing a meal four weeks previously.

He has been using salt water mouth washes in the hope the lesion would resolve spontaneously but as it is still present he has attended surgery seeking referral to ENT to have it removed; he is otherwise fit and well.

When you examine him you see this fluctuant swelling with a bluish translucent colour.

Which one of the following statements is incorrect?

A   This is an aphthous ulcer and should resolve within the next seven to ten days

B   This is a mucocoele and should be referred as it has not resolved of its own accord

C   Local trauma is a common triggering factor

D   Some may resolve spontaneously of their own accord

E   Some are chronic and require surgical removal; as they may recur, the adjacent salivary gland is excised as a preventive measure

F   They are more commonly found in children and young adults

45. Dermatology

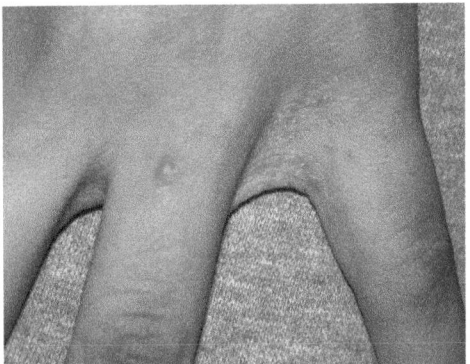

The wife of one of the officers at the local army barracks attends in a distressed state complaining of an intensely itchy rash over her body that started a few days ago; it is worse at night and despite changing her washing powder and shower gel it is getting worse.

You look closely and note burrows in between her fingers.

What is the name of the medication you will prescribe? ....

46. Dermatology: feet

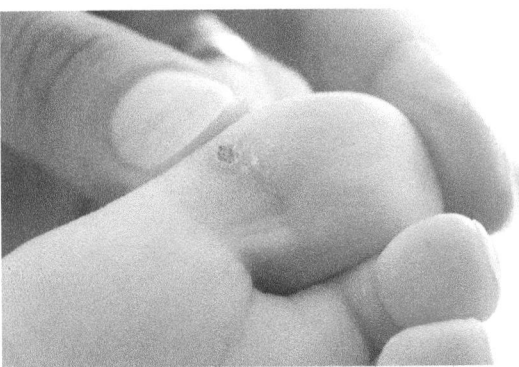

You see a 14 year old boy with this lesion on the sole of his left foot. *Which of the following options is the least cost-effective?*

A   Freezing
B   Diathermy
C   Salicylic acid
D   Duct tape
E   Surgery
F   Delayed immunisation with HPV vaccine

47. ENT

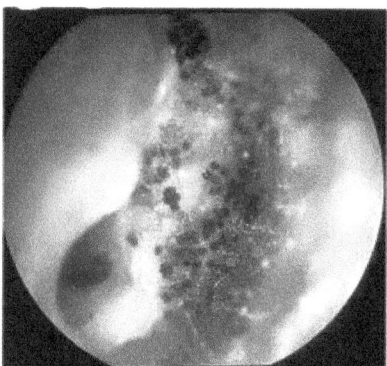

You see an otherwise healthy 52 year old lady with discomfort, irritation and discharge from her ear, having recently returned from a beach holiday. On examination her ear canal is moist and inflamed and you prescribe some antibiotic drops for a presumed diagnosis of otitis externa.

She returns ten days later requesting more drops as although her symptoms started to resolve, they have returned and she has terrible itching within the ear canal which is keeping her awake at night. On examination you see the above.

Which one of the following is the cause of this appearance and of her continuing symptoms?

A Allergic reaction to antibiotic drops
B Perforation of ear drum
C Fungal infection
D Debris and dried blood

Picture question answers 1-47

----

1. Answer D is true.

Shingles is due to re-activation of chicken pox virus; the rash is preceded by pain and the affected area is usually hyperaesthetic; the pain can be severe. It can occur at any age, but more commonly affects the elderly and immunocompromised.

Oral antivirals such as acyclovir are only effective if started within 48–72 hours of onset (*BNF* Sept 2007).

There is insufficient evidence to recommend topical lidocaine as a first-line agent in the treatment of post-herpetic neuralgia; it may benefit some patients but there is stronger evidence for use of other classes of drugs, e.g. gabapentin (Khaliq, Alam and Puri. Topical lidocaine for treatment of post herpetic neuralgia. *Cochrane Database of Systematic Reviews*, Issue 2).

2. Answer A is true.

An important study in the *Lancet* (2006; **367**: 397–403) showed that the classic symptoms of meningococcal disease presented late (median onset 13–22 hours); however, at a median time of 8 hours, 72% had developed early signs of sepsis (leg pains, etc.).

Penicillin i.m. should be given before urgent transfer to hospital (*BNF* Sept 2007).

Contact tracing and prophylaxis is undertaken by the local public health department.

3. Answer is E.

As the diamond does not cross the line of no effect, this meta analysis would indicate that circumcision may be beneficial in reducing the risk of syphilis, chancroid and genital herpes.

4. Answer is C.

If the confidence interval of the result, i.e. the horizontal line, crosses the vertical line of no effect, that can mean either there is no difference in outcome as a result of the intervention, or, that the sample size was too small for us to be confident of where the true result lies.

5. Answer is D.

The line of no effect as shown here is associated with a relative risk of 1.0.

6. Answer is A.

Each trial is represented by a line.

The area of the square is proportional to the statistical strength of the evidence in the study. The more subjects in the study, the larger the square.

7. Answer is E.

CSM advice in *BNF* (Sept 2007) is that oil and oil-based preparations such as vaseline and petroleum jelly are likely to cause damage to condoms and contraceptive devices made of rubber, making them less effective as a barrier method of contraception and as a protection from STDs including HIV; KY jelly is a non-spermicidal water-based lubricating agent that does not affect the latex; women should be advised to use spermicidal cream/pessaries with their diaphragms.

The *BNF* also states that clotrimazole cream can affect latex condoms/diaphragms.

8. Answer is D.

The child is presenting with leucocoria (white pupillary reflex); childhood leucocoria must be referred urgently as it may be due to retinoblastoma, a life-threatening tumour of early childhood. Prognosis is dependent on early detection and can range from cure to death. It may be hereditary or sporadic.

9. Answer is D.

The photo shows a picture typical of dry age-related macular degeneration with drusen affecting the macula.

10. Answer is A.

ST elevation in the anterior leads indicates that this man is having an acute anterior MI.

11. Answer B is true.

Bell's palsy is a lower motor lesion affecting the facial (seventh) cranial nerve; the whole of the side of the face is affected; the frontalis muscle is not spared as it is in an upper motor neurone lesion, e.g. CVA. The facial nerve supplies taste fibres to the anterior 2/3 of the tongue via the chorda tympani.

In herpes zoster oticus (Ramsay Hunt syndrome) severe pain in the ear precedes the facial nerve palsy; zoster vesicles appear in the external ear canal and on the soft palate.

12. Answer is A.

Peutz–Jeghers syndrome is characterised by mucocutaneous dark freckles on lips, oral mucosa, face, palms and soles (look closely at the hands!); it is autosomal dominant; there are benign intestinal polyps as part of the syndrome which can bleed or cause obstruction; malignancy occurs in 3%.

13. Answer is D.
These are milia; small white raised spots that are commonly seen in the neonate; reassure the mother that they will resolve on their own and that no treatment is required.

14. Answer B is true.
This patient is showing classical signs of rheumatoid arthritis with swelling of the fingers, metacarpal joints and ulnar deviation; RA is a chronic disease with a female : male ratio of 2 : 1 which affects not just the synovium joint but numerous other organs (pericarditis, pleurisy, anaemia, vasculitis, eye involvement, Felty's syndrome, etc.).

Research has shown that early diagnosis and treatment can improve disease outcome and early data have shown that if inflammation can be suppressed (by disease-modifying anti-rheumatic drugs, or, even more efficiently, by biological agents) at onset of disease, therapy can be withdrawn; the patient is in 'remission'. Many autoimmune diseases are positive for rheumatoid factor; it can also be found in the blood of 'healthy' asymptomatic individuals; it is sensitive but not specific for RA; anti-CCP antibodies are more specific (95% compared to 85%) (*BMJ* 2006; **332**:152-155; *Ann Intern Med* 2007; **146**:797-808).

15. Answer is B.
The picture is of erythema multiforme with its typical target or iris lesion; it may be related to his previous (presumed) strep throat or to penicillin, if he was prescribed this; it is usually self limiting and requires only symptomatic treatment; a severe form, Stevens–Johnson syndrome is more serious.

- Erythema nodosum: painful, raised red lesions on shin fronts.
- Vitiligo: white patches.
- Erythema ab igne: chronic inflammation, hyperpigmentation due to repeated exposure to external heat source, e.g. shins of elderly patients, as a result of sitting too near to fire.
- Erythrasma: infection by *Corynebacterium minutissimum*, intertriginious areas (groin, axilla) – brown discolouration may be treated with erythromycin as the drug of choice; but can use other antibacterial and / or antifungal agents.

16. Answer is E.
This baby has a strawberry naevus, also known as a capillary haemangioma; they are very common and the mother should be reassured that although the mark will get larger as the baby grows, it will start to regress of its own accord after the age of 3 or 4.

17. Answer is A.

Can be due to infection, sudden loud noise, barotrauma, insertion of sharp objects into ear; usually heals on its own; may need ENT referral if not healing, or if perforation is large, for tympanoplasty; advise patient to avoid getting water in – e.g., no swimming or diving; protect ear with cotton wool/ear plugs while showering/bathing, until healed.

18. Answer is A.

In diabetics, the most common cause of a vitreous haemorrhage is leakage from new vessels in proliferative retinopathy; central retinal artery thrombosis also presents as acute, painless partial visual loss, often in diabetics and hypertensives, but the retina is extremely pale, whitened by the ischaemia, except for a cherry red spot at the fovea where the retina is much thinner and the choroid shows through; acute glaucoma is painful. In hysterical blindness the fundus appears normal.

19. Answer is A.

The *BNF* (Sept 2007) states that although both terbinafine and (pulsed courses of) itraconazole have replaced griseofulvin for the treatment of onychomycosis, terbinafine is considered the drug of choice; mild localised infections may respond to topical therapy.

20. Answer is B.

Molluscum contagiosum is caused by a wart virus and, although it is very infectious, the government's HPA (Health Protection Agency) specifically advises that it 'isn't a serious condition and probably not highly contagious in schools .... no exclusion from school, work or swimming pools is necessary ..... although common sense measures such as avoiding sharing towels .... may reduce transmission'.

21. Answer is E.

This man has gout; oral NSAIDs are recommended for first-line treatment (Jordan *et al. Rheumatology*, 2007; British Society for Rheumatology and British Health Professionals in Rheumatology Guideline for the Management of Gout); colchicine is an effective alternative but is slower to work than NSAIDs; allopurinol should not be commenced during the acute attack.

There is evidence that obesity is linked with gout (e.g. Sutaria *et al. Rheumatology*, 2006; **45**: 1422–31); however, weight loss should be gradual and starvation or high protein diets which can elevate urate levels should be avoided. Thiazide diuretics aggravate gout and a medication review to change this to another anti-hypertensive should be considered.

22. Answer is A.

White patches on the tympanic membrane in someone with a long history of local infection (and/or trauma, e.g. grommets), are likely to be calcium deposition; if severe they can cause a conductive hearing loss; these deposits should not be removed as there is danger of perforating the ear drum.

23. Answer is A.

The patient has right bundle branch block, which although it is found in heart disease, can be a normal variant in otherwise healthy patients.

24. Answer is B.

Seborrhoeic warts are seen frequently in the elderly, especially on the chest; flat-topped, stuck-on appearance; benign; no treatment necessary unless bothersome.

25. Answer is A.

Basal cell carcinoma is the commonest malignant skin tumour; classically it has a pearly nodule with a rolled edge and surface telangiectasia; local invasion can be very destructive but metastases are rare. Occurrence predominantly on face and other sun-exposed areas.

26. Answer is E.

Squamous cell carcinoma – locally invasive and metastasise to local lymph nodes; can present as keratotic lump, a rapidly growing polypoid mass or, as seen here, a cutaneous ulcer; again, sun-exposed sites, especially lips. Also related to pipe and cigarette smoking.

27. Answer is C.

Malignant melanoma is the most dangerous of malignant skin tumours; occur in younger patients, incidence increasing; malignant melanoma can arise in pre-existing melanocytic naevi.

28. Answer is D.

Keratoacanthoma, rapidly growing lesion – enlarges over 6–8 weeks; round tumour with rolled edges and a prominent keratin plug; ultimately shrinks away leaving a small puckered scar.

Keratoacanthoma is also regarded in the dermatology community as a squamous cell carcinoma as it can behave in exactly the same way and the histology can be almost identical. For the purposes of management, keratoacanthoma should be managed as a squamous cell carcinoma.

29. Answer is F.

Kaposi's tumour, purplish plaques and nodules; classically in Ashkenazi Jews and northern Italians; more aggressive form seen in AIDS.

30. Answer is B.

This baby has cradle cap; management depends on severity but involves reassuring mum that the scaly rash will settle spontaneously in due course. In the meantime mum should apply baby shampoo / baby oil; if the rash becomes more severe, she could try a mild topical steroid (1% HC).

 Note that dermatology is considered a 'bread and butter' aspect of general practice and has been highlighted in the new national RCGP curriculum.

31. Answer is B.

This shows the lacy striae typical of lichen planus. Drugs that can cause lichenoid reactions include allopurinol, some ACE inhibitors, colloidal gold, some beta blockers, some oral hypoglycaemics, some NSAIDs, methyldopa, and antimalarials.

32. Answer is D.

Lymphoedema is the result of disturbance to the normal lymphatic flow, resulting in oedema of the limb; it can be uncomfortable for the patient and carries increased risk of becoming infected.

33. Answer is A.

34. Answer is B.

The audiogram in a patient with early noise-induced deafness demonstrates particular loss around 4000 Hz which is quite characteristic and sometimes described as a notch. With continued exposure to noise the sensitivity at 8000 Hz is lost as well.

35. Answer is C.

If there is a problem with the cochlea or the auditory nerve, the AC and BC thresholds will be the same.

36. Answer is D.

Glue ear results in conduction deafness. The pure tone audiogram shows hearing loss particularly at low frequencies and also bone conduction is higher than air conduction.

37. Answer is A.

Picture questions 38–41: In Rinne's test the vibrating tuning fork is placed over the mastoid process behind the ear to test bone conduction (BC). The patient indicates when he no longer hears the vibrating fork, after which the tuning fork is placed in front of the ear and the patient asked if he can hear it (air conduction = AC).

Weber's test consists of placing a vibrating tuning fork over the middle of the forehead; the patient indicates if the sound is louder in one ear than the other. With conductive hearing loss, from middle ear disease or obstruction of the external auditory meatus with wax, BC will be greater than AC and Weber's test will lateralise to the deaf ear. However, with sensorineural hearing loss AC is better than BC and Weber's test will lateralise to the good ear.

A patient with a very severe unilateral loss on the right, i.e. a dead ear, may be Rinne negative in the right ear with Weber lateralising to the left ear. In this case, Rinne's result is a false negative. On testing the right ear, the bone conduction is heard in the normal left cochlea by skull crossover.

Note: when there is suspicion of hearing loss, audiometry should be performed even if bedside tests are normal.

38. Answer is B.

39. Answer is C.

40. Answer is E.

41. Answer is F.

42. Answer is B.

Most likely Maisey will be four years old.

From the age of two to four most children tend to scribble; from the age of four to six most children start producing 'tadpole' drawings (large heads with legs and arms sticking out) and then progress to stick figures where there is a separate head and torso.

From the age of seven children usually produce much more detailed pieces with a strong narrative element.

43. Answer is A.

Nasal polyps can be distinguished from the inferior turbinate by their lack of sensitivity, their yellowish-grey colour and, if you are experienced in nasal examination, by your ability to get between them and the side wall of the nose.

Polyps are unusual in children so if they present, think of cystic fibrosis.

Nasal polyps tend to be bilateral. With unilateral lesions, suspect a tumour (and in children, rule out an encephalocele).

A foreign body would usually cause a unilateral, blood-tinged discharge, especially in young children.

44. Answer A is incorrect.

45. Answer is: permethrin dermal cream 5%.

Permethrin 5% dermal cream is the treatment of choice in the UK for scabies.

46. Answer is E.

Most plantar warts will resolve spontaneously if left alone, but patients do present for a number of reasons; in some areas treatment has now been banded as 'low priority' and patients may be advised to self-treat; surgery is not routinely recommended as there is no guarantee that the verruca will not return.

In a recent *BMJ* article (*BMJ* 2011; **342:** d3271), salicylic acid and cryotherapy were equally effective for clearance of plantar warts.

There has been some anecdotal evidence but no clinical trials to address the use of the vaccines in this area.

(*Gynecol. Oncol.* 2007; **107(2)(suppl 1):** S31–S33; *Arch. Dermatol.* 2010; **146:** 475–7).

47. Answer is C.

This appearance is typical of fungal infection which can sometimes occur after antibiotic / steroid treatment. Antifungal drops will usually settle the problem down (*BMJ*, 2012; **344:** e3623).

Appendix

Photograph permissions

Picture question 1
Reproduced from the National Library of Medicine.

Picture question 2
Reproduced courtesy of The Meningitis Trust
(www.meningitis-trust.org).

Picture questions 3–6
Image is reproduced from *Sexually Transmitted Infections*, 2006; **82**:101-10; courtesy
of the BMJ Publishing Group.

Picture question 7
Photo is reproduced with permission from Island Sexual Health
(www.islandsexualhealth.org).

Picture question 8
Reproduced with permission from the University of Michigan Kellogg Eye Center
(www.kellogg.umich.edu).

Picture question 9
Constable IJ. Age-related macular degeneration and its possible prevention. *MJA*,
2004; **181**: 471-72. © 2004, *The Medical Journal of Australia* – reproduced with
permission.

Picture question 10
© Brodie Paterson 2004. Reproduced from www.rcsed.ac.uk.

Picture question 12
Reproduced from www.ferengi.com.ar.

Picture question 13
© Crown copyright [2000–2005] Auckland District Health Board.

Picture question 14
Reproduced from www.arthritis.co.za.

Picture question 15
© Johns Hopkins University; reproduced from Withybush General Hospital PGMC
website (www.pdt-tr.wales.nhs.uk).

Picture question 16
Reproduced from www.baby-medical-questions-and-answers.com with permission.

Picture question 17
© 2007 Clinical Skills Education Centre, Queen's University Belfast.

Picture question 18
Reprinted with permission from eMedicine.com
(available at www.emedicine.com/emerg/TOPIC789.HTM [accessed 1 July 2013]).

Picture question 19
© www.curefootpain.co.uk – reproduced with permission.

Picture question 20
Reproduced from www.scienceblogs.com.

Picture question 21
Reproduced from www.flickr.com – photo by "mobiledoc".

Picture question 22
© 2007 Kevin T. Kavanagh; reproduced from www.entusa.com.

Picture question 23
Reproduced with permission from *The Merck Manual of Diagnosis and Therapy*,
Edition 18, edited by Mark H. Beers. © 2006 by Merck & Co. Inc., Whitehouse Station,
NJ. Available at www.merck.com/mmpe.

Picture question 24
Image courtesy of www.skinsight.com.

Picture question 25
Image courtesy of www.virtualmedicalcentre.com.

Picture question 26
© 2008 Memorial Sloan-Kettering Cancer Center. Reproduced from www.mskcc.org
with permission.

Picture question 27
© 2003–2008 Dermatology Online Atlas. Reproduced from www.dermis.net.

Picture question 28
© 2007 Dermatology.co.uk. Reproduced from www.dermatology.co.uk with
permission.

Picture question 29
© 2006-07 University of Washington. Reproduced from HIV Web Study,
www.hivwebstudy.org.

Picture question 30

© 2009 Bauer London Lifestyle. Reproduced from www.askamum.co.uk.

Picture question 31

© 1996–2009 C. Stephen Foster MD. Reproduced from www.uveitis.org with permission.

Picture question 32

Reproduced with permission of Dr Stanley G. Rockson (available at http://stanfordhospital.org/cardiovascularhealth/lymphaticvenous/).

Picture questions 33, 35 and 36

Reproduced under the Open Government Licence from www.dwp.gov.uk/ publications/specialist-guides/medical-conditions/a-z-of-medical-conditions/ hearing/tests-hearing.shtml.

Picture question 43

Reproduced with permission from www.entsheffield.co.uk.

Picture question 44

Reproduced with permission from www.doctorspiller.com.

Picture question 45

Reproduced from northampton.gp-surgery.com.

Picture question 46

Reproduced with permission from www.akronics.com.

Picture question 47

Reproduced with permission of Department of Otolaryngology, Head and Neck and Skull Base Surgery, St Vincent's Hospital, Sydney, Australia (available at http://sydneyentclinic.com).